the Beck
DIET
solution

train your brain
to **think** like
a thin person

the **Beck**
DIET
solution

train your brain
to **think** like
a thin person

Judith S. Beck, Ph.D.
Beck Institute for Cognitive Therapy and Research

Foreword by Aaron T. Beck, M.D.

Oxmoor
House®

Published by Oxmoor House, an imprint of Time Inc. Books,
a division of Meredith Corporation,
225 Liberty Street, New York, NY 10281

ISBN-13: 978-0-8487-3275-2
Library of Congress Control Number: 2006935166
Printed in the United States of America
Fourth Printing 2018

Be sure to check with your health-care provider before making any
changes in your diet.

Editorial and Production Support: Allison Long Lowery, L. Amanda Owens,
Melissa Jones Clark, Julie Boston, Laura Lockhart, Tamara Nall

To my husband

Contents

The Power of Cognitive Therapy for Weight Loss

The Program

chapter 5

Week 1: Get Ready: Lay the Groundwork   53

chapter 6

Week 2: **Get Set: Prepare to Diet** 96

chapter 7

Week 3: **Go: Start Your Diet** 140

chapter 8

Week 4: **Respond to Sabotaging Thoughts** 178

chapter 9
Week 5: **Overcome Challenges** 206

chapter 10
Week 6: **Fine-Tune Your New Skills** 238

Going Forward

Acknowledgments

Special thanks to Phyllis Beck and Naomi Dank, two remarkable women whose continual encouragement, advice, and support allowed me to write this book. And to Debbie Busis, who helped me develop and implement this program. Many thanks, too, to Richard Busis and Alice Beck, for their careful editing and helpful suggestions.

I would also like to thank the many people who inspired, informed, and produced this book: Sarah Busis, Ruth Hanno, Lois Whitman, Barbara Whitman, Jody Beck, Jane Hausner, Brian Carnahan, Beth Grossman, Mary Guardino, Mickey Stunkard, and the Beck Institute staff.

I am deeply grateful to my gifted editor, Alisa Bauman, who helped shape and translate my vision, and to Debora Yost, who helped sharpen my writing. And many thanks to my extraordinary agent, Stephanie Tade, who saw promise in a manuscript and was instrumental every step of the way in turning it into this book.

Thanks, too, to all the dieters with whom Debbie Busis and I have worked and from whom we've learned so much. And my deep gratitude to and overwhelming pride for my dad, Aaron T. Beck, M.D., whose development of Cognitive Therapy produced a revolution in the field of mental health.

Foreword
A New Application of Cognitive Therapy

There is a serious and growing health crisis in the United States. Nearly two-thirds of adults, and an ever-increasing number of children and adolescents, are overweight. And research continues to show that people who are significantly overweight are at higher risk for a number of diseases and medical conditions. Most individuals who lose weight on a diet start to gain it back within a year. Few medical treatments have been developed to ameliorate this problem, and the treatments that do exist have significant drawbacks. Medication can be effective in the short run but is accompanied by undesirable side effects. It's also short-lived: People tend to gain weight once they stop taking it. Bariatric surgery for severe obesity, as with any operation, carries risk and requires that patients eat drastically reduced portions of food (usually tablespoons at a time).

The Beck Diet Solution was developed to help provide an answer to this health issue. It contains the missing ingredient lacking in other weight-loss programs. Based on the techniques of Cognitive Therapy, it helps you learn to think differently so you can change your eating behavior—not just in the short run, but for the rest of your life.

Research shows that people can learn to change their behavior and, importantly, maintain the change. Battling spouses, for example, can learn how to communicate more effectively. Shy people can learn how to be more assertive. But unless they also change their thinking, they generally revert to their old behavioral habits sooner or later. The same kind of relapse is true in dieting. Unless you change your thinking, you won't be able to sustain new eating habits.

Dr. Judith Beck has created a novel step-by-step program that has a dual focus on changing both behavior and thinking. Most dieters know that they need to eat nutritiously, lose weight slowly, make dieting a priority, use good eating habits, be assertive with food pushers, tolerate hunger and craving, exercise, refrain from emotional eating, and motivate themselves continually. But they either don't know how to do these things or they don't know how to consistently get themselves to do these things.

When I first developed Cognitive Therapy as a treatment for depression, I had no idea that a whole new generation of psychologists and psychiatrists would apply this treatment to a wide range of psychiatric disorders, psychological difficulties, and behavioral health problems. Although the specific techniques vary somewhat from one problem to another, what remains constant across treatments is a focus on helping people to change their self-defeating thinking and beliefs. When people learn to think more realistically, they feel better and can achieve their realistic goals. Depressed patients, for example, have negative thoughts about themselves, their worlds, and their futures, which not only make them feel miserable but interfere with their daily living. Anxious patients overestimate the danger in various situations and, thus, feel nervous much of the time.

Dr. Judith Beck has identified the key distortions in the negative thoughts of dieters that prevent them from reaching and maintaining their desired weight. She has identified the crucial "sabotaging thoughts" of dieters. Examples are: Rationalizations (*It's okay to eat this because ...*); underestimation of consequences (*It won't matter if I eat this*); self-deluding thinking (*Since I cheated a little, I might as well eat whatever I want for the rest of the day*); arbitrary rules (*I can't waste food*); mind-reading (*My friend will think I'm rude if I don't eat her cake*); and exaggeration (*I can't stand being hungry*).

Learning how to correct these distortions, learning how to solve diet- and non-diet-related problems, and learning how to motivate oneself to adopt helpful eating behaviors is what distinguishes Dr. Judith Beck's program from all others. She developed the Beck Diet Solution over two decades, learning from her psychiatric patients who wanted to lose weight—and from her own experience as well.

It is with great pride that I wholeheartedly endorse this book. My pride is both professional and personal, since Judith is my daughter. I speak objectively, however, when I say that she is not only a world expert in Cognitive Therapy, but also a gifted therapist, supervisor, and teacher. In addition to writing more than 50 articles and chapters on a variety of applications of Cognitive Therapy, she has also written several books, including the basic textbook in our field that has been translated into 18 languages and is used worldwide. She has presented hundreds of workshops and trained thousands of people in Cognitive Therapy, both nationally and internationally. I predict that her latest contribution to the field, *The Beck Diet Solution,* will have a profound impact on people who wish to lose weight.

Aaron T. Beck, M.D.
University Professor of Psychiatry
University of Pennsylvania
School of Medicine

Introduction

I'm so glad that you've chosen *The Beck Diet Solution* to help you lose weight and keep it off. I developed and fine-tuned this program during the many years I've worked as a Cognitive Therapist.

It's been wonderful working with dieters during the past 20 years. It's been so gratifying to see how their lives have improved; how losing weight built their confidence; and how their confidence helped them to form new relationships, get better jobs, and engage in more enriching activities. Equally important, losing weight has helped them improve their health, feel better physically, and improve their quality of life.

Although each dieter I've counseled had a slightly different story, all of them had struggled to lose weight, sometimes since their teen years. But it hadn't been for lack of trying. They had all lost *some* weight—but every one of them had gained back most, if not all, of that lost weight. Why had they been so unsuccessful?

These dieters thought they hadn't been able to lose weight or keep it off because they were weak or didn't have enough willpower. But these explanations just weren't true. They hadn't lost weight or kept it off because they didn't know *how.* They didn't know how to motivate themselves continually. They didn't know what to do when they were tempted to cheat. They didn't know how to view their slips as temporary mistakes, not as signs to give up. They didn't know what to do when they felt overwhelmed, hopeless, or unable to keep going. They didn't realize that they could learn how to diet successfully, just as they had once learned to drive a car or to use a computer.

They also didn't know that dieting has many natural ups and downs. For many people, dieting is relatively easy at the beginning. And then, at some point, they meet their first challenge, and dieting gets hard. This happens to everyone. Yet, once the dieters I've counseled learned to expect these rough patches—and to plan for them ahead of time—they were able to persevere and get through these temporary difficulties. I equip the dieters I counsel with many preparatory tasks and skills—before they ever start dieting. This preparation teaches them exactly what to do when dieting gets hard.

The Beck Diet Solution prepares you in the same way. You'll be able to face challenges with confidence because you'll know exactly how to get through them, and each time you do, dieting will become easier and easier.

The difficulty and frequency of these challenges will gradually diminish until eating differently is just a way of life.

I'd like to start you off on your weight-loss journey with some wisdom from people who have faced rough patches in dieting and gotten through them. I recently asked dieters I'm working with to list what they know now about dieting that they wish they'd known years ago. This is what they said:

I now know …

- I can control my eating if I plan in advance what I need to do and if I practice what I need to say over and over to myself.
- when I'm tempted to eat something I shouldn't, I need to pull out my list that contains all the reasons I want to lose weight.
- just because I'm hungry doesn't necessarily mean I should eat.
- cravings always go away, and there are things I can do to make them go away faster. I don't have to give in to them.
- eating a reasonable breakfast and lunch is important so I won't overeat at night.
- if I don't follow a nutritious diet, I'm more likely to cheat.
- I have to make time for dieting and exercise.
- I have to prepare in advance for sabotaging thinking.
- I need to sit down and eat slowly and notice every bite—every time I eat.
- if I eat something I shouldn't, it's just a mistake. It doesn't mean I'm hopeless or bad. I don't have to make it a bigger mistake by continuing to eat whatever I want for the rest of the day.
- I have to put my needs first sometimes.
- it's okay to say no to people who offer me food.
- I have to watch out for fooling myself. Every single time I put food in my mouth, it matters.
- I need to give myself credit every time I do what I'm supposed to do.
- if I regain weight, I can go back to using the skills I learned to lose it—every time.
- I can do it! I have the skills now. I know how to do it, and I'll have these skills forever.

If I'd told these dieters—at our first sessions—that they would one day make these statements, they wouldn't have believed me. You, too, might not believe it at first, but one day soon you will. Slowly, step-by-step, the Beck Diet Solution will build your confidence. When you finish the program, six weeks from now, revisit this page and look at this list of bulleted statements. You'll realize that you agree with every one of them. And you'll also realize that—this time—your weight loss will be permanent.

The Power of Cognitive Therapy for Weight Loss

chapter 1

The Key to Success

If you've had difficulty losing weight or have lost weight in the past only to gain it back, did you blame yourself (*I'm too weak ... I'm not motivated enough*), your body (*There's something wrong with me ... I just can't lose weight*), or your diet (*This just didn't work for me*)?

I'm happy to tell you that there's a completely different reason that you haven't been successful. You just didn't know *how* to diet. Once you know *how* to diet, you'll step on the scale and see a lower number reflected week after week after week. You'll drop clothing sizes. You'll experience all the wonderful benefits that come along with a slimmer body: more energy, more confidence, better health, and improved self-esteem, as well as fewer aches and pains. You can have all of this—and continue to have it for a lifetime. It doesn't ever have to slip away from you as it may have in the past. You can end the weight loss–regain cycle—*permanently*.

You can do all this once you learn how to continually follow a diet. The Beck Diet Solution teaches you *how* to avoid cheating; *how* to resist tempting food, even if it's on the table right in front of you; and *how* to cope with hunger, cravings, stress, and strong negative emotions without turning to food for comfort. You'll also learn *how* to motivate yourself to exercise, even if you're not naturally inclined to do so. You'll discover how to do all the things you need to do to diet successfully—by *changing the way you think.*

Most dieters who end up in my office have been on and off diets for years. They all have one thing in common: They don't know how to think like a thin person. People who struggle with weight loss have a mindset that sabotages their efforts. For example, they often have such thoughts as:

- *I know I shouldn't eat this, but I don't care.*
- *It's okay if I eat [this food] just this one time.*
- *I've had such a hard day. I deserve to eat this.*
- *I can't resist this food.*
- *I'm upset. I have to eat.*
- *I ate something I shouldn't. I may as well blow my diet for the rest of the day.*
- *This is hard. I don't want to keep dieting.*
- *I'll never lose weight.*

If any of these thoughts sound familiar to you, you're the perfect candidate for the Beck Diet Solution. This program teaches you how to talk back to your sabotaging thoughts in a convincing way. When you hear that little voice in your head say, *Oh, just eat it ... It won't matter,* you'll be able to tell yourself, *Yes, it* does *matter ... I want to be thin ... Every time I eat something I'm not supposed to, it makes it more likely that I'll give in again in the future ... It matters every single time ... I'm just trying to fool myself ... If I eat it, I'll get a few seconds of pleasure, but then I'll feel bad ... I can resist this ... I want to lose weight much more than I want a few seconds of pleasure.*

no more "cheating"

The word *cheat* doesn't appear again in this book outside of this box. I've omitted it intentionally because too many unsuccessful dieters have all-or-nothing thoughts about their eating: *Either I'm perfect on this diet or I've cheated ... If I've cheated, I've blown it—I may as well continue to cheat for the rest of the [day/week/month/year].* I've found that people who view themselves as having cheated usually feel demoralized and even "bad," which makes it even more difficult for them to get back on track.

Instead of *cheat,* I've used the words *unplanned eating* and *overeating.* These terms are less negatively charged. People who use them are able to take a more benign view and say, *Okay, so I ate something I didn't plan to eat or I ate more than I was supposed to.* But they're also able to then add, *It was just a mistake, no big deal ... I'll get back on track for the rest of the day.*

If you're ambivalent about starting the Beck Diet Solution, consider this: Many people gain a few pounds every year due to a natural age-related slowing of the metabolism. Add to this the fact that it takes only 20 or so extra calories a day to gain 2 pounds a year. This means that if you're 10 pounds overweight today and do nothing about it, a year from now you may be 12 or 13 pounds overweight ... the year after that, perhaps 14 or 15 pounds ... and so on and so on. But instead of gaining, you can lose weight and maintain your weight loss by practicing the principles you'll learn in *The Beck Diet Solution.*

Any reasonable diet will work for you if you have the right mindset.

The Beck Diet Solution is a psychological program, not a food plan. It doesn't tell you *what* to eat—you can choose any nutritious diet you want. That's because any reasonable diet will work for you if you have the right mindset. The Beck Diet Solution teaches you how to get yourself to eat the way you're supposed to eat. It shows you how to talk back to the *I don't want to, I don't have to,* or *I can't* voice in your head.

To choose appropriate foods and to use appropriate eating behaviors consistently and permanently, you have to learn how to make permanent changes in your thinking. With the comprehensive, step-by-step program in this book, you'll be able to stay on your diet, lose weight, and maintain your weight loss for life.

The Power of Cognitive Therapy

The Beck Diet Solution is based on the principles of Cognitive Therapy (also known as Cognitive Behavior Therapy, or CBT), the most highly researched and effective form of talk therapy in the world. My father, Aaron T. Beck, M.D., spurred a revolution in the field of mental health when, in the late 1950s and early 1960s, his research challenged the theories of Sigmund Freud. Freud and his followers believed that depression and other types of mental illness stemmed from a patient's repressed fears and conflicts, and they kept patients in daily psychoanalytic sessions over a period of years.

My father discovered, however, that depressed patients could get better quickly—often with just 10 or 12 sessions of therapy. When he helped his patients set goals, solve problems, and change their depressed thinking, their depression quickly abated. Because a major component of the treatment focused on correcting people's distorted thinking, he called this new form of treatment "Cognitive Therapy." The word *cognitive* refers to thinking.

In the ensuing years, my father and researchers all over the world adapted Cognitive Therapy for many different psychological disorders and problems. Hundreds and hundreds of research studies have demonstrated that it helps people with a wide range of difficulties, including depression, anxiety, eating disorders, obesity, smoking, and addictions. Even more impressive, people not only get better, but also they *stay* better. They learn how to change their inaccurate, unhelpful thinking in order to feel better emotionally and behave in more productive ways to reach their goals.

A recent study in Sweden demonstrated the effectiveness of Cognitive Therapy for weight loss. People enrolled in the Cognitive Therapy program lost an average of 18 pounds over 10 weeks of treatment. (Meanwhile, people on a waiting list to get into the program didn't lose *any* weight.) But here's the truly impressive part: When the study participants were evaluated a year and a half after their treatment, nearly all of them—92 percent—had not only maintained their weight loss, but also most had lost even more weight. This is what sets Cognitive Therapy apart from other types of therapy and other types of weight-loss programs.

Compare this result with people who diet but don't receive Cognitive Therapy treatment. Research completed at Tufts University found that between 50 to 70 percent of people who started one of four widely used diets were unable to stay on their diets and continue to lose weight for a year. Even more discouraging, other studies that track how people fare after they lose weight reveal a sobering trend: Most people who lose weight on any given diet regain most of the lost weight within a year.

How Cognitive Therapy Works

Cognitive Therapy is based on the concept that the way people think affects how they feel and what they do. For example, let's say you have the thought *I'm hungry*. If you then have "sabotaging thoughts"—such as,

Cognitive Therapy helps you
*identify your sabotaging thinking and
effectively respond to it,* so you feel better
and can behave in helpful ways.

This is terrible ... I can't stand it ... I have to eat!—you'll feel panicky and grab some food. On the other hand, if you counter your thought with "helpful responses"—*But it's all right ... I'm going to eat in a couple more hours ... I can wait*—you'll feel in control and get involved in an activity. Cognitive Therapy helps you identify your sabotaging thinking and effectively respond to it, so you feel better and can behave in helpful ways.

Cognitive Therapy teaches people how to solve problems, and dieters can have lots of problems. For example, have you ever strayed from a diet for any of the following reasons:

- You finished all of the food on your plate but didn't feel satisfied.
- You felt upset and thought that eating would make you feel better.
- You were too tempted by the sight of food when shopping at the supermarket.
- You were too tired to cook, so you opted for fast food instead.
- You were too polite to turn down the dessert that your friend baked.
- You were at a party and felt like treating yourself.

To successfully lose weight and keep it off, you need to solve these kinds of practical problems. You'll also need to solve some psychological problems, such as:

- Feeling overwhelmed by the requirements of your diet
- Feeling deprived
- Feeling discouraged when you don't lose weight consistently or lose as much weight as you had hoped
- Feeling stressed by other life problems

Cognitive Therapy helps you solve both practical and psychological problems and learn new thinking and behavioral skills—skills you'll be able to use for the rest of your life. You'll not only overcome your current problems, but also learn how to use your new skills to overcome future problems.

Are You Like Sue?

For more than 20 years, I've used Cognitive Therapy to help many people resolve many different problems, including struggling to lose weight. Sue* is typical of these dieters. Before Sue came to treatment, she'd tried many diets, off and on, ever since high school, only to become mired in a familiar cycle: During the first few weeks or months of each diet, she'd confidently lose weight and feel in control; eventually, however, something would make her stray.

*The names of all dieters in this book have been changed.

The reasons varied. One day her boss asked her to work late, which, she said, "caused" her to pick up a pizza on the way home. Another time, after an argument with her husband, she was upset and "found" herself eating a pint of chocolate ice cream. Yet another time she "lost control" at a holiday party while at a buffet table covered with one tempting dish after another.

Whenever Sue gave herself an excuse to deviate from her diet, her resolve quickly diminished. She'd continue to eat out of control. Then she'd feel like a failure, decide she'd never be able to lose weight, and give up entirely, eventually gaining back all the weight she'd lost—and sometimes more.

Sue began yet another diet soon after her first session with me. The first two or three weeks of her new diet went smoothly, but then she had a setback. She was so upset by a situation at work that she began "to eat everything in sight." Fortunately, Sue came to see me the next day. When we examined what Sue had eaten, it became apparent that she had not "totally blown" her diet. I helped her see that if she just got right back on her diet, she would likely gain, at most, a half pound for the week—*not* a major setback. By changing her thinking from, *I'm such a failure ... I'll never be able to lose weight,* to *I can start again right this moment,* she was able to get back on track.

Sue continued to have some mild setbacks along the way, but she learned how to keep these setbacks in perspective. She also learned how to prepare in advance for stressful times. She got to the point where she was able to stick to her plan, no matter what was going on in her life. She broke out of her yo-yo dieting cycle, lost more than 55 pounds, and has kept it off for more than 12 years.

Sue's story is typical of the dieters I work with now and have worked with over the years. It can be your story as well.

Whether you're depressed or content,
a stay-at-home or working parent, a binge eater or
social eater, a dieting novice or dieting pro,
the Beck Diet Solution can help you.

No Lost Causes

The Beck Diet Solution is based on the same plan that I use with my patients who want to lose weight. It works, regardless of your unique psychological makeup, lifestyle, and family circumstances. Whether you're depressed or content, a stay-at-home or working parent, a binge eater or social eater, a dieting novice or dieting pro, this program can help you.

In the past, you may have been able to make short-term changes in your eating habits to help you lose weight. But when the going got tough, you abandoned those changes because you didn't know how to talk back to such sabotaging thoughts as:

- *Dieting is too hard!*
- *I have to eat this. I have no self-control.*
- *I don't want to hurt her feelings, so I'll eat what she made.*
- *I can't diet when I'm stressed.*

The set of psychological strategies in this book will help you in many ways. You'll learn how to resist the urge to overeat when you're confronted with cravings, hunger, stress, social pressures, and myriad other problems. You'll learn how to follow your diet and exercise programs no matter what happens. You'll learn how to think like a thin person. These strategies take practice, but in time they'll become automatic.

My Story

I personally can understand the challenges that dieters face, and I also can attest to the success of using Cognitive Therapy to overcome them. I started dieting as a teenager and went on and off diets for many years. I, too, had lots of sabotaging thoughts, such as:

- *I should eat as little as possible.*
- *If others don't see me eating, it doesn't really count.*
- *If I give in to temptation, it's my fault for being weak.*
- *If I eat something I hadn't planned to eat, I may as well abandon my diet for the whole day.*

How did I finally succeed at losing weight and keeping it off? I learned from patients I counseled. One of the first people I worked with when I became a psychologist was a woman who suffered from depression and anxiety. After several weeks of therapy, she began to feel better and told me she had a new goal: She wanted to lose weight. Well, it was easy for me to see how unrealistic and inaccurate *her* thoughts were when it came to eating and dieting. I could readily see how *she* needed to change her thinking so she could change her eating behavior. I learned a lot from her and from many subsequent patients who also wanted to lose weight. Then I applied what I had learned to myself, and I lost 15 pounds. That was many years ago, and I've kept it off ever since.

During the past 20 years, I've learned through trial and error what works and what doesn't. During this time, I discovered a number of crucial factors. For example, I've found that to lose excess weight and keep it off, it's important to do the following:

- Choose a nutritious diet.
- Create time and energy for dieting.
- Plan what and when you're going to eat.
- Seek support.
- Deal with disappointment.
- View overeating as a temporary problem that you can solve.
- Cope with hunger and cravings.
- Eliminate emotional eating.
- Give yourself credit.

You don't yet know how to do all these things—or how to get yourself to continually do these things—but you will.

With the Beck Diet Solution, you'll learn one new skill every day. By the end of six weeks, you'll have learned everything you need to continue losing weight and to be on your way to keeping it off—permanently.

You'll get to the point where you react differently when you see food you know you shouldn't eat.

The New You

You'll probably find that dieting and weight loss follow a predictable cycle: During the first week or two, you might find that dieting is relatively easy. Then things likely become somewhat more difficult. Cravings set in or intensify. Life intervenes. Your schedule gets busy. You feel emotionally stressed. And you might come up with any number of reasons to stray from your diet.

If you just keep practicing the skills described in this program, however, you'll do fine. Dieting will become easier. Cravings and hunger will diminish. You'll learn better ways to deal with stress. Your thinking will change. In fact, you'll get to the point where you'll react differently when you see food you know you shouldn't eat. Instead of saying, *I wish I could eat this,* and feeling sad, or *It's unfair that I can't eat this,* and feeling unhappy, you'll automatically say, *I'm so glad I'm not eating that.* At some point, you'll shift from, *I hate depriving myself,* to *I'm happy I didn't overeat!* Just take it one day at a time, as this book suggests. You'll get there!

the solution at a glance

- Cognitive Therapy is a psychological treatment that will help you successfully lose excess weight and keep it off.
- The way you think about food, eating, and dieting affects your behavior and how you feel emotionally.
- Certain ways of thinking make it difficult to follow a diet and to maintain weight loss.
- The Beck Diet Solution takes you through a six-week process to change sabotaging thoughts (that cause you to stray from your diet) to helpful thinking (that will lead to success).

chapter 2

What *Really* Makes You Eat

D o you ever feel as if you eat automatically, that eating is some-how out of your conscious control? Many of the dieters I've worked with certainly have felt this way at times.

Well, the good news is that your eating is *not* automatic. Automatic processes are involuntary, such as the beating of your heart or the digestion of your food. You don't *decide* to let your heart beat or to set off your digestive processes. You *do* decide to eat, however. And here's the other good news: You can *learn* how to take better control of your eating decisions.

The Thought Comes First

You may not be conscious of it, but you always have a thought before you eat. Let's say you see an open package of peanut butter crackers on the counter. You don't just automatically reach for a cracker and put it in your mouth. Your *thoughts* influence what you do. If you think, *I really want to eat that ... It won't matter if I take one,* and you don't respond to those thoughts, you'll go ahead and eat the cracker. On the other hand, if you think, *I really want to eat it, but I shouldn't because it's not on my diet ... I have to get better at resisting food between meals,* then you won't eat it.

The thoughts that lead you to act in unhelpful ways are sabotaging thoughts. The thoughts that lead you to act in more productive ways are helpful thoughts.

Here is how Jim's thoughts influenced his eating behavior. Before I started working with him, Jim often frequented an Italian restaurant that served really great bread. Even though he was trying to diet, he would invariably have such thoughts as, *The bread smells so good ... I know I shouldn't eat it, but I just can't resist.* So, of course, he would end up eating a piece. Then he would have the thought, *I've blown it ... Oh, well, I might as well start again tomorrow.* And he would overeat for the rest of the meal.

A few weeks after we began working together, Jim had plans to go to the same restaurant. But this time, he was prepared to answer his sabotaging thoughts. Before he went, he wrote and read a card that said:

> Remember, the bread will be tempting, but I *can* resist it. It's more important to me to lose weight. If I eat the bread, I'll get momentary pleasure, but afterwards I'll feel worse.

Jim, indeed, was tempted to eat the bread. He did have the thought, *That smells so good, I really want it.* But this time he was able to respond to his sabotaging thought. He didn't give himself the choice to take any bread. He was really pleased by this accomplishment.

You can learn to do what Jim did.

How Thoughts Can Sabotage Your Diet

Sabotaging thoughts make dieting more difficult in many ways:

Sabotaging thoughts encourage you to eat. You'll probably notice that you have a number of "permission-giving" thoughts that allow you to rationalize what you eat. These thoughts often start with the phrase, *I know I shouldn't eat this, but it's okay because....* They end with any number of excuses, such as, *I had a hard day ... This is a celebration ... It will just go to waste ... I really want it ... It won't matter.* And so on, and so on, and so on.

Sabotaging thoughts undermine your confidence. These are the thoughts you have after you've eaten something that you think you shouldn't. For example, instead of just saying to yourself, *Okay, I made a mistake ... I shouldn't have eaten that, but I can start eating in a better way right now,* you say, *It's so terrible that I ate that ... I'm so weak ... I'm just not going to be able to lose weight.*

These are also the kind of thoughts you might have when you see the scale go up, even though you've been eating properly. Instead of saying to yourself, *Okay, no big deal ... I should just keep on doing what I've been doing and the scale will probably go down next week—and if it doesn't, I can solve the problem then,* you say to yourself, *This is terrible ... This is never going to work ... I may as well give up now.*

Sabotaging thoughts allow you to disregard the advice in this book. As you read various parts of *The Beck Diet Solution,* instead of thinking, *I should really carry out every task in the program so I'll have the greatest chance of success,* you might think, *I don't really have to do [this task].* For example, you might think, *I don't have to write down what I'm eating ... I can remember without writing it down.* Or, *I don't have to sit down when I eat ... I like eating while I'm standing up.*

Sabotaging thoughts increase your general level of stress. Dieting takes time and energy, so it's important to reduce your overall stress whenever you can. The way you think about non-dieting-related situations can either increase or decrease your stress. For example, instead of thinking, *I'm just human ... It's okay to have strengths and weaknesses,* you might think, *I should always do things perfectly.* This kind of thinking increases your general level of stress because perfection is not attainable. Instead of thinking, *I should generally try to be a nice person if I reasonably can,* you might think, *I should always make everyone happy.* This is another highly stressful idea because it also represents an impossible goal.

Throughout *The Beck Diet Solution,* you'll learn how to identify and respond to all of these kinds of sabotaging thoughts.

If you can *identify the triggers that evoke sabotaging thoughts* and lead you to eat in unhelpful ways, you can *minimize your exposure to them* or *change your response to them.*

which muscle are you strengthening?

Throughout the pages of *The Beck Diet Solution,* you'll find that I often refer to two "muscles": your resistance muscle and your giving-in muscle. I'm actually talking about your tendency to think and act in certain ways.

Every time you resist eating something you shouldn't, you're strengthening your tendency to resist in the future. However, each time you give in and eat something you shouldn't, you're strengthening your tendency to give in.

So whenever you feel the urge to eat something you're not supposed to, think about which muscle you really want to strengthen. If you want to lose weight and keep it off permanently, you need to take every opportunity to strengthen your resistance muscle and to weaken your giving-in muscle.

Eating Begins with a Trigger

Sabotaging thoughts arise when you're confronted with a trigger, a situation that stimulates your thinking. You're probably most aware of *environmental triggers,* such as seeing or smelling food. You can also experience *biological triggers,* such as hunger, thirst, or cravings (intense urges to eat).

There are also *mental triggers:* thinking about food, reading a description of food, recalling something you enjoyed eating (or a situation in which you didn't eat and felt deprived), or imagining eating food in the future.

Then there are *emotional triggers.* These are unpleasant feelings, such as anger, sadness, anxiety, frustration, or boredom. You eat to comfort or distract yourself. Emotional triggers can also be pleasant feelings. You might think that if you eat or keep eating, you can keep that good feeling going. Or you might eat because you think your good feeling will go away if you restrict yourself.

Finally, there are *social triggers.* Examples include people who urge you to eat or situations in which you want to be able to eat like everyone else.

If you can identify the triggers that evoke sabotaging thoughts and lead you to eat in unhelpful ways, you can minimize your exposure to them or change your response to them. The Beck Diet Solution shows you how to deal with triggers by learning how to do the following:

- Modify your eating environment.
- Tolerate hunger and craving.
- Think differently about food.
- Deal with your emotions in a productive way.
- Make eating healthfully a higher priority than pleasing other people or satisfying a momentary desire.

Many people who struggle to lose weight think they're hungry when they're not.

There are differences between hunger and other sensations that masquerade as hunger. The Beck Diet Solution shows you how to differentiate between the triggers described below so that you can make appropriate decisions about eating.

Hunger: You experience an empty sensation in your stomach, which is often accompanied by stomach rumblings.

Thirst: You feel a dry sensation in your mouth when you have a need to take in liquid.

Desire: You want to eat because of another trigger (frequently environmental), even if you've just eaten.

Cravings: You have a strong urge to eat a certain kind of food, which is accompanied by tension and an unpleasant yearning sensation in your mouth, throat, or body.

From Trigger to Eating

Sometimes, the chain of events that ends in eating is straightforward:

You encounter a trigger: Someone offers you a piece of cake.

You have a thought: *That cake looks good.*

You make a decision: I think I'll have it.

You act: You eat the cake.

At other times, the chain of events that ends in eating is a little more complicated. You strongly argue with yourself before you make the decision to eat. You think to yourself, *I think I'll have it ... No, I really shouldn't ... But I really want it ... It's not on my diet ... It looks so good ... But I'm not supposed to eat it.* Depending on where this inner argument ends, you either make the decision to eat it or you make the decision not to eat it.

This inner argument between your sabotaging and helpful thoughts can make you feel tense. The tension is unpleasant. Often, you'll try to alleviate that tension by deciding to eat. But before you eat, take note: Interestingly, what usually happens is that you find your tension abating as you reach for the food—*before* you put it in your mouth. However, just as the decision to eat can reduce tension, the decision *not* to eat can also reduce tension.

The Beck Diet Solution teaches you how to effectively respond to the sabotaging thoughts that lead to inappropriate eating. It's a skill you'll need not only to lose weight, but also to keep excess weight off permanently. If you've never been taught this skill, it's no wonder you either had trouble losing weight or always regained it in the past. You'll use this skill into the future, whenever you have sabotaging thoughts, as Emma's story illustrates below.

> ## Just as the decision to eat can reduce tension, *the decision* not *to eat* can also reduce tension.

A Great Example of Helpful Thinking

Emma had lost more than 40 pounds when I counseled her many years ago. I hadn't heard from her in more than 10 years when she called to say hello. She told me that she had maintained her weight loss with comparative ease. I asked her if she still had sabotaging thoughts and, if so, what she did about them. Emma thought for a moment and gave me the following example: About two weeks prior to the phone call, Emma was tempted by sticky buns that someone had left on the counter in the office kitchenette. Most days, she would have ignored them completely, but she was particularly hungry that day. She knew if she tried to eat just a small piece of this high-fat, high-carbohydrate food, she would want more. During the next few hours, she had lots of thoughts: *I'm hungry. They look so good. I'd really like to have one.* Fortunately, she was well equipped to answer these thoughts each time one occurred:

- *No, I don't need to eat them. I'm having lunch in two hours. Leave the kitchenette.*
- *No, I don't need to eat them. I just had lunch a couple of hours ago. If I hadn't come in here to get a cup of coffee, I wouldn't even have thought about them. Get my coffee and leave.*
- *No, I don't need to eat them now. I'm avoiding making a phone call. Go do it or find something else to do.*
- *No, I don't need to eat a sticky bun, even though I'm really hungry. This hunger will go away soon if I concentrate on my work. And, besides, it's not that long until dinner.*

Emma also positively reinforced herself every time she refrained from eating the sticky buns. She didn't say, *Darn, I wish I could eat them.* She said, *That's great that I didn't eat them.* In this way, she strengthened her resistance muscle and weakened her giving-in muscle.

If you've never had the experience of feeling proud of yourself for not eating, you're in for a wonderful surprise. Keep reading and do all the tasks in the Beck Diet Solution program. You'll not only lose weight, but also you'll be so glad that you learned how to control your sabotaging thinking so you can permanently control your eating.

the solution at a glance

- Eating is not automatic. You *can* learn how to take control.
- Many situations trigger thoughts about eating, but there are techniques that you can learn to avoid or minimize these triggers.
- When you encounter a trigger, your thoughts determine whether you act in a productive way that strengthens your resistance muscle or in an unproductive way that strengthens your giving-in muscle.
- Responding to your sabotaging thoughts is a skill that you can use for your lifetime to keep off excess weight permanently.

chapter 3

How Thin People Think

Have you ever wondered why you can't lose weight or keep off the weight you've lost? You certainly know many people who don't struggle with eating the way you do. Are you different? You probably are, but not necessarily for the reasons you think. Consider the following questions:

- Do you sometimes eat even when you're not really hungry? In other words, can you easily tell the difference between being hungry and just wanting to eat?
- Are you sometimes concerned that you might not have an opportunity to eat? Do you ever have such thoughts as, *What if I get hungry later?*
- Do you sometimes eat past the point of mild fullness?
- Do you fool yourself about your eating? In other words, do you sometimes tell yourself that it "won't matter" if you eat a small piece of something you're not supposed to eat?
- Do you comfort yourself with food?
- If the scale goes up, do you sometimes abandon your diet altogether?
- Do you sometimes eat because it doesn't feel fair that you can't eat just like everyone else?
- Do you stop dieting as soon as you've lost weight?

If you answered yes to any of these questions, then you possess characteristics that can make dieting difficult.

characteristic 1

You Confuse Hunger with the Desire to Eat

Naturally thin people are more easily able to differentiate between when they're truly hungry because their stomachs are empty and when their stomachs aren't empty but they have a desire to eat.

Thin people say to themselves, *I know I'd like to eat [that food] ... But I just ate a little while ago ... I'm not going to have it*. You, on the other hand, may label any desire to eat as hunger. You probably get the idea that you ought to eat whenever your stomach feels empty and you feel an urge to eat.

The Beck Diet Solution

To think like a thin person, you must learn to tell the difference between hunger and the desire to eat so that you can make better decisions about when it's appropriate to eat and when it's not. You'll do so by paying attention to how your stomach feels before and after meals. You'll also do such experiments as purposefully making yourself hungry so that you learn to recognize what true hunger feels like.

characteristic 2

You Have a Low Tolerance for Hunger and Cravings

Most thin people feel hungry and occasionally notice cravings, but they don't dwell on these feelings. Generally, they don't think that much about food at all. They figure they'll always be able to find something when they're hungry or be able to withstand the hunger if it's not convenient to eat. Usually, they have no problem holding off until their next snack or meal.

When you're hungry or have a craving, though, you might dwell on these feelings. You probably worry about when you're going to have an opportunity to eat again. Maybe you even become preoccupied with thoughts of food. You're likely to overestimate how strong your hunger and cravings will get and how long they'll last. It's likely you'll try to get rid of them right away by eating. In fact, some people who struggle to lose weight experience hunger and cravings as emergencies: *I must eat now!*

> To think like a thin person you must *learn to tell the difference between hunger and the desire to eat.*

The Beck Diet Solution

In this program, you'll discover for yourself that hunger and cravings are not emergencies, and you'll learn how to tolerate them. As you're reading this, perhaps you're thinking, *I know I don't have to eat when I'm hungry or having a craving ... I* want *to eat.*

You've probably read about hunger strikes, so you know people can go for days without eating. If you've ever fasted for a religious observance or a medical procedure, you know firsthand that hunger waxes and wanes.

Yet at the moment you feel hungry or experience a craving, you might not be thinking rationally. You might feel that you have to do something about it immediately to satisfy your urge to eat. Perhaps this inaccurate thinking stems, in part, from our hunter-and-gatherer ancestors, who survived only if they developed the ability to focus their attention intently on eating when food was around so that they could gain weight to survive leaner times when food was scarce. Today, food is plentiful all the time, but our modern brains have not yet caught up to this modern reality.

I'm going to teach you how to effectively respond to the voice in your head that tries to convince you, *I have to eat right now!* You'll learn many techniques to refocus your attention so that hunger and craving lose their persuasive power. You'll learn to tell yourself, *I'm just feeling hungry,* or *I'm just having a craving ... I don't have to pay attention to it ... I can shift my focus to something else ... I don't have to eat impulsively to get rid of this feeling ... In a few minutes, I'm going to be really glad that I didn't eat.*

characteristic 3
You Like the Feeling of Being Full

Thin people usually like to eat to the point where they're reasonably full. It doesn't feel right if they've eaten so much they feel a little uncomfortable taking a brisk walk after a meal. Even if there is delicious food left, they don't *want* to keep eating. They feel no compulsion to empty their plates.

You, however, might feel uncomfortable if you *stop* eating at that same point. There are three possible reasons you feel this way:

- One, you may be concerned that you'll get hungry again before the next meal.
- Two, you may feel deprived if you don't eat as much as you want.
- Three, you may have grown accustomed to eating much greater quantities than is healthy. Indeed, you may label the degree of fullness you feel after an overly large meal as "normal" when you've actually eaten to the point of overfullness.

I noticed this phenomenon recently when I had dinner at the house of a colleague. There were 10 of us in all. Although I'm usually oblivious to what people eat, on this particular night I decided to pay attention. This is what I observed: Two of us (both women) ate sparingly. Three of the men (all of normal weight) ate more than we did, but not a great deal more. The other five (all of whom are overweight) ate much more than the rest of us.

We light eaters skipped the hors d'oeuvres and several of the side dishes altogether and ate some of the entrée, vegetables, and rice. The moderate eaters had some hors d'oeuvres and finished most of what was on their plates. The big eaters ate lots of hors d'oeuvres and side dishes and finished just about everything on their plates. They couldn't possibly have still been hungry, yet all of them had seconds. They also ate much larger portions of dessert.

Why did they eat well beyond the point of fullness? Probably because they all had such thoughts as:

- *This tastes so good. I don't want to stop.*
- *It's a special occasion, so it's okay to splurge.*
- *I want to show my hostess that I appreciate her efforts.*
- *I can't resist such wonderful food.*

They probably also overate because they *wanted* to feel overly full at the end of the meal.

The Beck Diet Solution
This program teaches you how to change your mindset so that you actually feel good about feeling reasonably full at the end of meals. It takes practice, but you'll get to the point where instead of feeling deprived when you get up from the table, you'll automatically say, *I'm so glad I didn't overeat.*

characteristic 4
You Fool Yourself About How Much You Eat

Thin people generally have a pretty good gauge of how much they eat. They don't overeat very often, and when they do, they naturally eat less at their next meal or two to compensate for it.

People who struggle with dieting, however, often delude themselves about how much they eat. In fact, at times you might deliberately try not to notice what you're eating because you know you would feel bad if you really paid attention. For example, you might eat a pint of ice cream standing at the freezer or finish an entire bag of chips while watching TV. It's as if part of you believes, *If I'm not fully conscious of what I'm doing, it's okay to keep eating.*

You'll learn how to effectively respond to the voice in your head that tries to convince you that you must eat right now!

You might tell yourself that what you're eating doesn't really matter—that is, the calories don't count if you're only eating the crumbs in the bottom of a bag of cookies, the icing that's left on the cake cutter, or a broken piece of pretzel. Maybe you justify eating too much because you're eating out, celebrating, or vacationing. Or you might make the excuse that you should eat something because it's free or someone is urging you to eat.

You can also fool yourself in other ways. You might use eating something that you shouldn't have as an excuse to eat even more. Perhaps you've said to yourself, *Since I strayed from this diet, I may as well blow the whole day.* So you eat and eat, promising yourself you'll start again tomorrow.

could you have an eating disorder?

If you jump from diet to diet without being able to sustain your weight loss, you're an excellent candidate for the Beck Diet Solution.

If you have an eating disorder, however, you'll need professional help that is beyond the scope of this book. To make sure you don't have an eating disorder, answer the following questions:

• Do you have a continuous obsession with food, dieting, weight, or appearance to the exclusion of more important aspects of your life?

• Do you already weigh in the lower range of what is considered your ideal weight? (If you don't know what your ideal weight is, ask your health-care provider.)

• Do you have a history of severe food restriction?

• Do you frequently binge-eat and purge—that is, deliberately vomit after eating—or abuse laxatives?

• Do you severely overdo exercise to try to keep your weight down?

If you answered yes to any of these questions, please make an appointment with a mental-health professional. This program is not suitable for you. In addition, if you have a health problem, make sure your health professional thinks it's a good idea for you to diet.

The Beck Diet Solution

As you read this, you can probably see how this kind of thinking doesn't make good sense. Yet, in the moment, your sabotaging thoughts override your rational mind. Recognizing and responding in a helpful way to these sabotaging thoughts is a key component of this program. You'll be practicing this skill daily.

characteristic 5

You Comfort Yourself with Food

When thin people are emotionally upset, they don't turn to food for distraction or solace. It just doesn't cross their minds. If anything, they tend to lose their desire to eat.

On the other hand, when you're distressed or bored, you might immediately want to grab food. Eating can distract you from your negative feelings and soothe you. In fact, there are certain foods—chocolate, for example—that contain substances that release "feel good" chemicals in your brain.

The problem, of course, is that you feel better only momentarily. What happens as soon as you're finished eating? You still have to deal with the problem that made you upset. And, on top of that, you feel bad that you strayed from your diet. You become self-critical, undermine your confidence, and feel even worse than you did at the start.

The Beck Diet Solution

Instead of trying to comfort yourself with food, the Beck Diet Solution teaches you to calm down in other ways: by using distraction and relaxation techniques, by countering your sabotaging thoughts, and by solving the problems that were associated with your negative emotions in the first place.

characteristic 6

You Feel Helpless and Hopeless When You Gain Weight

When thin people gain weight, they don't usually see it as a catastrophe. They figure that they'll simply watch what they eat for the next few days or increase their exercise. They have confidence that the scale will go back down.

You're probably different, though. What goes through your mind when you see on the scale a higher number than you'd expected? You probably

*The Beck Diet Solution teaches you
how to* learn from your eating mistakes and
to recommit yourself *to your diet right away.*

have such thoughts as, *I can't believe it! This is terrible! I'll never lose
weight!*

Thin people have faith in their ability to make good decisions about
what, when, and how much they're going to eat—and to follow through
with these decisions. Even when they eat more than usual, such as at a
party, they're confident that they'll return to a more controlled way of eating afterwards.

You, however, may have constant sabotaging and demoralizing thoughts
that undermine your confidence. When you overeat, you might believe
that you'll never be able to control your eating.

The Beck Diet Solution

This program teaches you many techniques to prevent overeating. But,
equally important, it also teaches you how to learn from your eating
mistakes and to recommit yourself to your diet right away. When you do
so, your confidence grows. You'll know that you can immediately recover
from slips and control your eating and weight.

characteristic 7

You Focus on Issues of Unfairness

Are you surprised to learn that most thin people restrict their eating to
some degree? They might be trying to maintain their weight or to stay
healthy—or both. So they sometimes eat smaller portions than they
would really like and choose healthy foods when they'd really prefer to
eat something else. They accept these limitations without too much
struggle. They just don't think about it very much.

You, however, might frequently reflect on how unfair it is that others
can eat what they want but you can't. Truth is, not only do you underestimate how much others restrict themselves, but also you overly focus
on the injustice you feel because you have to limit yourself. In the past,
this kind of thinking may have led you to stray from your diet, or you may
have given up your diet entirely.

Most thin people, especially women,
*stay thin by being incredibly careful about what
they eat.* They might tell you that they don't
work at it, but mostly they do.

The Beck Diet Solution

So many of the dieters I've worked with were preoccupied with the unfairness of dieting that I decided to do an experiment, which turned out to be a lot of fun. I asked numerous people who don't struggle with dieting (they ranged from very thin to "normal" weight) if they would change their eating habits if all foods contained exactly the same number of calories and were equally nutritious. Many of them, especially men over age 40 and most women (of any age), told me that, yes, they would eat differently. Either they would eat certain foods more frequently or they would regularly eat larger quantities of food. In other words, they usually *do* restrict their eating.

I also came to the conclusion that there are two types of thin people: Those who don't have to work at staying thin and those who do. For the most part, those who don't have to work at it have small appetites, don't eat unless they're hungry, and get sufficient exercise. The rest fall into the second category: They have to work at it. Most thin people, especially women, stay thin by being incredibly careful about what they eat. They might tell you that they don't work at it, but mostly they do. This doesn't mean they're lying; they're just so used to eating the way they do, they consider it the norm. To them, eating small portions and lower-calorie foods is a way of life. They decide that fattening foods are either entirely out of bounds, or, more likely, they indulge in them only occasionally.

It's natural to look at some people and compare what they're eating to what you're eating—but it's not helpful. With the Beck Diet Solution program, you'll learn how to accept the restrictions you have to impose on yourself to reap the rewards of losing weight.

characteristic 8
You Stop Dieting Once You Lose Weight

There is a significant difference between people who have lost weight and kept it off for many years and people who constantly yo-yo diet (losing weight, regaining it, losing it, and regaining it). People who end up maintaining their new weight do so because they've changed what they do and how they think about food and eating. If you think that you'll be able to return to your old ways of eating after you lose weight, you'll gain the excess weight back.

The Beck Diet Solution

In order to lose weight this time, you'll learn crucial Cognitive Therapy techniques that you'll use for *the rest of your life*. They include planning what you eat, choosing healthy foods, resisting cravings, soothing yourself without turning to food, using good eating habits, and exercising, to name but a few. You'll also learn essential skills to counter sabotaging thoughts that would otherwise lead to overeating, demoralization, and giving up. And you'll learn how to *motivate* yourself to use your skills in the future.

The good news is that once you learn these skills, dieting becomes much easier. And so does maintaining your weight loss. The dieters I counsel tell me this all the time. It doesn't require as much effort to maintain your weight as it does to lose it—*if you learn the skills you need along the way.*

If you're struggling to accept the idea that you're going to need to make significant and permanent changes to your eating habits, you might benefit from reading this transcript from one of my sessions with Megan, a dieter who was grappling with the same issue.

Megan: I don't know. I just don't get it. You're saying that even after I lose weight, I still won't be able to eat whatever I want—for the rest of my life?

Dr. Beck: I bet that sounds pretty bad to you.

Megan: It does! I don't understand. I mean, I see people eating pizza and doughnuts and all kinds of stuff like that all the time! How come they can eat it and I can't?

Dr. Beck: I don't know the scientific answer. How many of these people have lost a significant amount of weight?

Megan: I don't know.

Dr. Beck: My guess is that they've always been roughly the same weight; they aren't trying to maintain weight that they've lost. Or maybe they're eating a lot at the moment but aren't eating like that during the rest of the day. Let me ask you this: Who do you know who has lost weight and kept it off?

Megan: Well, I know lots of people who've lost some weight, but they all gained it back. I know, my cousin Jennifer! She lost about 20 pounds a long time ago, and she hasn't gained it back.

Dr. Beck: Okay, think about Jennifer. Have you been to some family dinners with her in recent years?

Megan: Yeah.

Dr. Beck: How does she eat?

Megan: She's really careful ...

Dr. Beck: What does she do?

Megan: She doesn't eat that much. She's kind of particular. I noticed she always asks for salad dressing on the side, and she always just eats the main course. I know for a fact she doesn't eat dessert. Or bread.

Dr. Beck: Does she eat pizza and doughnuts and food like that?

Megan: I doubt it. Not very often, anyway.

Dr. Beck: The people you know who gained back weight—how careful are they?

Megan: Not very.

Dr. Beck: Is it possible that the people you see eating pizza and doughnuts are either not losing weight or not trying to keep it off?

Megan: I guess. But that's pretty discouraging.

Dr. Beck: Yes, it is, but I think you'll be so much less discouraged if you realize three things: One, you can always plan to have at least small portions of pizza and doughnuts if you want. Two, your craving for these foods is going to go way down. Three, the payoff for not eating these foods whenever you want them is huge. You've told me how important it is to you to lose weight.

Megan: Yeah, it is, but it's still disappointing to hear that I'll always have to watch what I'm eating.

Dr. Beck: Of course, it is. But what you don't know is how much less disappointed you'll be when you're maintaining a much lower weight and feeling good about yourself. My guess is your disappointment will be really minor and not very frequent. It won't be like it is today. You'll be at a restaurant or someone's house, everyone will be eating some fattening dessert, and you'll say to yourself, *You know, that looks good ... But how great is it that I don't feel compelled to eat it ... I'm much happier being thinner.*

the solution at a glance

- If you struggle with weight loss, you have a different mindset about food and eating than people who don't struggle with their weight.
- The way you think—seeing hunger as an emergency, overestimating the discomfort and duration of cravings, underestimating how thin people restrict their eating—makes it more difficult for you to stick with a diet.
- No matter what your mindset is like today, you can learn how to change it, not only to lose weight, but also to make sure that you keep it off—permanently.

chapter 4

How to Use the Beck Diet Solution

D uring the next six weeks, you'll begin to make over your mindset and, as a result, gain the skills you need to make over your body. You'll learn how to motivate yourself and how to feel good about eating differently. You'll develop a consistent sense of control that will continue to grow the longer you practice the techniques in this program. And you'll learn how to use your new skills for a lifetime, so you'll be able to maintain your weight loss.

I predict that six weeks from now, when you look back and compare yourself with how you are today, you'll be surprised at how much you've changed—and not only because you've lost weight. You'll realize that you're a different kind of eater. You'll have a full set of new tools and a new-and-improved mindset that will last forever.

A Program for Everybody

The beauty of the Beck Diet Solution is that it can help *anyone*. It doesn't matter if you want to lose 5 pounds or 100 pounds or if you just want to maintain your weight. It doesn't matter if you're male or female, old or young. It doesn't matter whether this is your first or tenth diet, or whether you've been dieting on and off forever. If you want to keep off excess

This program is designed to help you
solve the problems that have made dieting
difficult for you in the past.

weight permanently, you need to have a good set of dieting skills. All I ask is that you choose a healthy, nutritious diet (make sure to get approval from your health-care provider) and that you don't start dieting until you're psychologically ready, which might not be until two weeks from today.

Many dieters I've worked with over the years were initially a little hesitant about starting this program. It made sense to them, but they were concerned that it might be difficult, that it would take too much time, or that they wouldn't be able to stay motivated. They didn't realize that the program was designed to help them solve these very problems. They also didn't know (although they quickly found out) that dieting would become easier and easier as they learned and practiced the skills I was going to teach them.

Like those dieters, you might also feel hesitant. You might not believe right now that dieting will become easier—but it will. The Beck Diet Solution is designed to help you solve the problems that have made dieting difficult for you in the past.

The Two-Week Wait

Every diet provides you with a plan that tells you what you should and shouldn't eat. But knowing what to eat is only a small part of successful dieting. In fact, the Beck Diet Solution doesn't tell you what to eat. You can choose any reasonable diet. If you followed a sensible diet in the past but couldn't lose weight or keep it off, it wasn't necessarily the diet's fault. You just didn't have the skills to make the diet work—now, you will. This program teaches you how to eat, how to motivate yourself every day, how to create time and energy for dieting, how to solve diet-related problems, and how to use many other essential techniques.

If you've already taken a look at the Contents page or flipped ahead in the book, you probably noticed the program suggests you start your diet on Day 15. Why wait to start dieting? Because you need time to build the skills that will make your diet a success. During the first two weeks of this program, you'll learn and practice these skills. Some of the techniques are so effective that you might start losing weight even before you officially start your diet. In fact, researchers at the University of Pennsylvania reviewed a series of studies in which behavioral techniques were used instead of prescribing a diet. They found that participants were able to lose weight if they engaged in goal setting, problem solving, and self-monitoring (keeping a written log of what they ate). All of these skills are also incorporated in the Beck Diet Solution.

If you start dieting too soon—that is, before you have the skills you need—you might find dieting too challenging. You might get discouraged and maybe even abandon the program altogether. *Readiness is more complicated than simply wanting to change.* Think about other changes you've made in your life. For example, you didn't suddenly start driving one day simply because you wanted to. You had to learn driving skills one at a time. You had to practice them over and over until you got good at them and developed a measure of confidence in your ability to drive safely. It's the same with dieting. You need to learn certain skills and to develop confidence in your ability to use them consistently.

I encourage you to follow the program as written, by giving yourself a full two weeks to prepare. But I've worked with enough dieters to know that you might not want to wait that long. I also realize that you may have picked up this book because you're already on a diet and want to learn how to stick with it. Whether you decide to wait until Day 15, want to start dieting tomorrow, or are already dieting or maintaining your weight, you still need to prepare your mindset. Start on Day 1 and do each step in sequence.

A Task a Day

You'll have a new task to complete every day for the next six weeks. You'll perform some tasks only once. Others you'll do daily or weekly. The program is designed for you to progress one day at a time so that you can learn one skill before moving on to the next.

What if you feel very motivated and want to move more quickly? You can try this approach, especially during the first week of the program. For instance, you might be able to create your Advantages Response Card (Day 1 on pages 54–62), choose a primary diet (Day 2 on pages 63–69), and commit to eating sitting down (Day 3 on pages 70– 73) all at once. But, *most of the time,* you'll do much better if you stick to one day at a time. I don't want you to take on too much too soon and end up feeling overwhelmed. Err on the side of going slowly. It takes time to let new ideas sink in and to become proficient at changing your ideas and behavior.

On the other hand, if you find that one task a day is too much for you, implement changes more gradually. You can spend a week on each task, if needed. I don't mind how long it takes you to finish the program as long as you eventually do every step in order.

It takes time to let new ideas sink in
and to become proficient at changing
your ideas and behavior.

What You'll Need

Before you start the Beck Diet Solution, you'll need three inexpensive office supplies: index cards, sticky notes, and a bound notebook.

You'll use the index cards many times over the course of the program. You'll write important messages on them and read these messages to yourself several times a day. I suggest you use 3 x 5 cards because they're small and can fit into a purse, wallet, or pocket; if you prefer, you can use business-sized cards instead (available at office-supply stores). You'll also write reminder messages on sticky notes and put them in strategic places. The notebook is for keeping track of important diet-related information.

Looking Forward

If you follow the 42 steps in the six-week Beck Diet Solution program, you'll find that dieting is easier than it ever has been in the past. Like the dieters I've worked with in person, by e-mail, or over the phone, you'll discover the following things:

- Your cravings will diminish.
- You won't panic when you're a little hungry.
- You'll automatically plan what you're going to eat each day.
- You'll consistently follow your plan, even on special occasions.
- You'll feel good about turning down food instead of feeling deprived.
- You'll be proud of yourself.

And, of course, you'll be able to enjoy other benefits, too:

- You'll be thinner!
- You'll feel better about yourself.
- You'll be more confident.
- You'll have more energy.
- You'll feel better physically.

You'll also discover dozens of additional benefits as you lose weight and maintain your weight loss. All of these wonderful things were experienced by the dieters I've worked with—and they'll happen for you, too!

Many dieters tend to procrastinate. You, too, might have difficulty starting a diet because you continually tell yourself, *I don't think I'm ready ... I'll start another time.* Behind your reluctance might be a concern about failing. This transcript from a session with one of my patients might help.

Sandy wanted to lose weight, but she was ambivalent about starting a diet. Our discussion helped her realize that the stakes weren't as great as they seemed.

Sandy: I don't know. It just seems like this is going to be a lot of trouble.

Dr. Beck: You're right. It *will* be a lot of trouble.

Sandy: I don't know if I'm motivated enough to do it.

Dr. Beck: You may not be. Let me ask you, are you motivated enough to look at the advantages and disadvantages of starting the program?

Sandy: I guess so.

Dr. Beck: You don't sound very confident.

Sandy: I don't know. I have a lot of things going on in my life right now.

Dr. Beck: Is there any reason you should start the program now, as opposed to, say, a year from now?

Sandy: *[sighs]* I really don't want to be this heavy a year from now.

Dr. Beck: Are you sure? Sandy, it sounds to me like you're feeling pretty overloaded right now. Maybe what we need to do first is to unload some things. Once you're unloaded, you might be more ready to start the program.

Sandy: I don't know. Part of me really wants to start now. Part of me is a little scared to, I guess.

Dr. Beck: What's the scared part?

Sandy: What if I can't do it? What if I do follow the program and it doesn't work?

Dr. Beck: Well, what's the worst that would happen if you couldn't do it?

Sandy: I'd just quit, I guess. But I would be pretty disappointed.

Dr. Beck: So you might need to talk to me or to someone else about how to handle your disappointment, so you don't feel so bad?

Sandy: Yeah, I guess so.

Dr. Beck: If you decide to start dieting now, it's going to be important to realize that it's not so bad if you can't do it or if it doesn't work. You'll just have to go to Plan B. Try something else or try this program again later.

Sandy: Yeah.

Dr. Beck: So what do you think? How about if you don't start the program this week. Just think about whether or not you want to do it. Remind yourself that it's not such a big deal whether you start now or not, whether you can do it or not, and whether it works or not. You could always give it a try for about three weeks, if you want, and then decide whether or not to continue it.

Sandy: That sounds pretty good.

the solution at a glance

- You'll do a new task on each day of the six-week program.
- The tasks for the first two weeks will help you get ready for dieting.
- If you're already dieting or trying to maintain your weight, the skills in the first two weeks are still essential for long-term success.
- You'll need to purchase index cards, sticky notes, and a bound notebook.

The Program

chapter 5

Week 1

Get Ready: Lay the Groundwork

I know you may have had trouble losing weight in the past—but, if so, this time will be different. You're going to learn *how* to diet. During the next two weeks, you're going to learn crucial strategies that you'll need to diet successfully and to maintain your weight loss.

Throughout these two weeks, you'll use Cognitive Therapy techniques to prepare your mind and environment for dieting. This preparation will pay off when you successfully meet your first major challenge—and every challenge thereafter. The time you put into getting ready will help you to:

- Talk back to your sabotaging thoughts.
- Reduce the frequency and intensity of cravings.
- Remain motivated to follow your diet, even when you experience intense cravings.
- Be more conscious of every bite you eat.
- Increase your satisfaction during and after meals so you're less likely to reach for second helpings.
- Solve problems that have caused you to go off diets in the past.
- Feel more confident about your ability to follow your diet consistently, even when the going gets tough.
- Feel more accountable for every calorie you consume.

You'll use Cognitive Therapy techniques to *prepare your mind and environment for dieting.*

Many dieters overlook these important issues when they're trying to lose weight. They start dieting with no preparation. Don't make this mistake! I've found preparation is one of the most crucial components of dieting success.

Before coming to me, none of the dieters I counseled had spent time getting ready. They just picked a diet and started it that day. Guess what? They succeeded for a while, eventually faced a challenge, strayed from their diet, got discouraged, and quit. At some point, they got back on the same diet—or a different one—only to go through the identical sequence of events. Once I taught these dieters the essential techniques they needed, dieting went much more smoothly. They still faced challenges, but their preparation made these challenges surmountable. No matter what happened, they were able to follow their diet, lose weight, and keep it off.

And you can do the same.

What if you've already lost weight? You *still* need to prepare. Start with Day 1 and progress from there. Practicing the skills in this program is crucial to maintaining weight loss. It's insurance that all your hard work will pay off for a lifetime.

day 1

Record the Advantages of Losing Weight

Today, you'll make your first Response Card, an essential tool that will help you change your mindset and overcome the sabotaging thinking that interferes with losing weight. Response Cards are index cards (or the equivalent) that contain important written messages to help you counter your sabotaging thoughts. They also help you motivate yourself every day so that you can stick to your diet, apply good eating habits, deal with hunger and cravings, resist emotional eating, and get right back on board when you make mistakes.

You'll read these cards daily as you lose weight—and periodically for the rest of your life. They are an essential part of the Beck Diet Solution program. Chances are, you've never created, much less read, cards like these. No wonder hunger and craving have gotten the better of you in the past!

The card you create today might be the most important one of all. On it, you'll list the reasons you've decided to diet. Right now, I'd like you to think of all of the advantages of losing weight and *write them down* while they're clear in your mind. I want you to read this Advantages Response Card (or cards, if your reasons don't all fit on one) every day.

Now that you know what you're supposed to do, are you thinking, *Why write the reasons down? I'll always remember why I want to lose weight.*

It might seem hard to believe that you could ever forget these reasons. But, believe me, it's easy to forget when there's tempting food around. There'll be plenty of times when your resolve will falter and you'll have sabotaging thoughts, such as:

- *Is dieting really worth it?*
- *Resisting this food is too hard.*
- *I don't think I really want to do this.*

Do you remember having thoughts like these before? If so, you know just how persuasive they can be. Chances are, there were times when you bought into these kinds of thoughts, strayed from your diet, and stopped losing weight—or, worse, quickly gained back the weight you had worked so hard to lose. You need to learn how to combat these kinds of sabotaging thoughts in a strong, forceful way. Otherwise, you might very well follow your old path of giving up when the going gets tough.

If, on the other hand, you read your Advantages Response Card several times a day, every day, these reasons will be firm in your mind when you're tempted to eat something that you shouldn't. You'll be able to remember why you want to lose weight at the very moment your sabotaging thoughts are desperately trying to convince you that it's okay to eat something you know you shouldn't. You'll be able to say to yourself, *As much as I want to eat [this food] and enjoy a moment or two of pleasure, losing weight is much more important to me.*

You'll start making Response Cards now, on Day 1, because reading them is an essential strategy for lasting weight loss. Creating your first card should take you less than 10 minutes, and it should take you less than a minute to read this card each day.

Benefits of Weight Loss

So, why *do* you want to lose weight? Take a moment to think about this question. How will weight loss impact the following?

- Your love life, friendships, family, career, and social life
- Your energy level and participation in hobbies and recreational activities
- Your body, health, self-image, and mental outlook

Losing weight will likely affect them all for the better, but I'd like you to think about each of these specifically. For example, losing weight might mean feeling comfortable undressing in front of your partner. It might mean getting back to tennis, golf, dance, or other recreational activities you once liked but now find too physically taxing. It might mean enjoying outings to the beach or to social functions without worrying about how others think you look.

Try to think of as many advantages as you can. As you start to lose weight, you'll undoubtedly discover additional benefits along the way. For example, you might feel more confident and do things you don't usually do, such as speak up at meetings or volunteer to join a committee. Write the advantages on an index card and continue to add to this list any time you come across a new advantage you hadn't previously included.

To get started, consult the Reasons I Want to Lose Weight Chart on the facing page. This list of advantages comes from dieters I've counseled in my practice. I think many of the reasons will strike a chord with you.

Please *do not skip* this important exercise. It's not optional. Check off all the items that apply and write in your additional reasons; then rate them as instructed. It's important to do this now before reading further.

Finished? Okay, now you're ready to create your first card (or cards).

As you start to lose weight, *you'll undoubtedly discover additional benefits* along the way.

extra advantages

There are four *major* benefits to dieting that may not have occurred to you:

1. Your cravings will diminish.
2. You won't struggle over whether or not to eat something you know you shouldn't.
3. You'll feel good when you resist unplanned eating.
4. You won't feel guilty and demoralized because you gave in to cravings.

You may not believe right now that you'll achieve these things. But if you follow this program, you'll get to the point where you find that you just don't argue with yourself over what to eat and what not to eat. It'll be second nature for you to say no to food that's now difficult to resist. Can you imagine how wonderful it will be when this happens?

Reasons I Want to Lose Weight Chart

Check off all of the advantages that apply to you. Use the four additional blank spaces at the bottom to fill in others that are more specific to your life. Then, at the right of each advantage, rate how important each is to you: somewhat important, important, or very important.

Advantages to Losing Weight	How Important This Advantage Is to Me
○ I'll look better.	
○ I'll be more attractive to others.	
○ I'll be able to wear a smaller size.	
○ I'll be able to wear more stylish clothes.	
○ I'll be happier when I look in the mirror.	
○ I'll get joy out of shopping for clothes.	
○ I won't feel so self-conscious.	
○ I'll get more compliments.	
○ I'll be in better health.	
○ I'll be able to exercise without discomfort or embarrassment.	
○ I'll live longer.	
○ I'll feel better physically.	
○ I'll have more energy.	
○ I'll be more physically fit.	
○ I'll enjoy sexual intimacy more.	
○ I'll like myself more.	
○ I'll feel more in control.	
○ I'll feel as if I've accomplished something important.	
○ I'll have more confidence.	
○ I'll increase my self-esteem.	
○ I'll be less self-critical.	
○ I'll feel more outgoing.	
○ I'll do more things (like go to the beach).	
○ I won't have to listen to my family comment about what I'm eating.	
○ I'll be able to be more assertive.	
○ I won't mind eating in front of others.	
○ I won't have anyone bugging me about my weight.	
○	
○	
○	
○	

Make Your Advantages Response Card

Copy all of the advantages you've identified onto a 3 x 5 index card (or the equivalent) so that you can carry them around in your appointment book, wallet, purse, or pocket. You're going to read this card at *least twice a day* until you no longer struggle with dieting—and then whenever the need arises.

To make the list more compelling, itemize the advantages in order of importance to you. Copy your reasons verbatim from the Reasons I Want to Lose Weight Chart (page 57) or express them in your own words. If a reason is personal and you don't want to risk others seeing it, write it down in a code that only you will understand.

If you prefer, use business-sized cards and write just one reason per card. Or write or type the reasons on a piece of paper. Do whatever works for you. Just remember that you'll need to carry this list with you because you'll need to read it at various times during the day.

Check out the front and back of the card Carol, a dieter I counseled, made:

Advantages Response Card

1. I'll look so much better.
2. I won't be so self-conscious all the time.
3. I'll be able to wear clothes I like.
4. I'll feel in control.
5. I'll be able to move around better.
6. I won't feel embarrassed at the swimming pool.
7. I'll feel more confident.
8. I'll be happier when I look in the mirror.

9. My doctor won't bug me.
10. Sharon will be proud of me.
11. I'll be happier when I step on the scale.
12. I'll be able to wear my old clothes.
13. I'll look better for John's wedding.
14. I'll have more energy.
15. My sister won't make comments.
16. I'll feel better in my body.
17. My back won't hurt so much.
18. I'll feel better about myself.

In addition to carrying your card(s) with you, you might want to put the list in other places you'll often see it. Dieters I've counseled came up with these creative ideas:

- Turn the list into a screen saver for your computer.
- Program your e-mail to send items from your list as pop-up messages at regular intervals throughout the day.
- Copy the list on sticky notes to put on the bathroom mirror, refrigerator, or car dashboard.
- Post the list on the inside cover of your diet notebook.

Use Your Advantages Response Card

When and how you read your Advantages Response Card is important, since it will help you strengthen your motivating voice and weaken your sabotaging voice. There are two circumstances when you'll need to read your card:

1. Daily, at scheduled times. Read your card at least twice a day, at specific times—exactly when is up to you. You might find reading it before meals helps you stick to your eating plan. You also might decide to read it during typically difficult times of the day when you have trouble controlling your appetite; for many people, this is in the hour before lunch, in the late afternoon, and/or in the middle of the evening.

2. Whenever you find yourself struggling with cravings, temptation, or sabotaging thoughts. Some days, you might only need to pull out your card at scheduled times. Other days, when cravings are stronger, you might find yourself pulling it out repeatedly. For example, many dieters I counsel find that they need to review it more frequently on weekends and holidays than on weekdays.

Using your card effectively requires that you do more than simply read the words. Every time you read an advantage, think to yourself, *How important is this to me?* Rating each benefit in this way makes you think more carefully than if you simply allow your eyes to quickly glance at the words. This active process of reflection further helps you internalize these reasons and commit them to memory, allowing you to answer your sabotaging voice whenever it tries to convince you that it's okay to stray from your diet.

Remember to Read Your Advantages Response Card

Until reading your card becomes a habit, you might need a reminder system. You can do several things: Put a copy of the card itself or a sticky note reminder in places where you know you'll easily see it, perhaps on your car dashboard, office desk, bathroom mirror, refrigerator, or computer screen. The reminder might read, "Read Advantages Response Card" or "Read ARC."

You can set your watch, cell phone, personal digital assistant (PDA), or computer to sound an alarm at the relevant times. You can move your watch or a bracelet to the wrist you don't normally wear it on. The unfamiliar feeling will cue you to pull out the card. Right now, I'd like you to think of a reminder system. Make sure to put it into action before the end of the day.

Motivate Yourself to Read Your Advantages Response Card Daily

There might be times when that little voice in your head says, *You don't have to read your card … Everything is under control.* This is just another example of sabotaging thoughts getting in your way. You might even need a card to encourage you to read your Advantages Response Card, such as:

I need to read my Advantages Response Card at least twice a day if I want to resist temptation. It'll take only a few seconds. It's not a big deal. I might not need it psychologically today, but I'll need it soon. I have to cement these reasons in my mind for when the going gets tough.

Face Reality!

Did you read on to this part of the chapter without creating your Advantages Response Card? Please don't fool yourself that you can skip this step. If you want to lose weight permanently, you have to change the way you think about eating, dieting, and yourself. If you follow only some of the steps, you'll probably have trouble losing weight or maintaining your weight loss. Then you'll blame yourself: *I just can't do this! I can't lose weight!*

Think about it: If your doctor gave you an antibiotic to get rid of a bad infection, would you take only half the pill? Of course not. Likewise, don't take shortcuts with this program. It's most effective if you follow it in its entirety.

Your Advantages Response Card is the first of many Response Cards you'll create to answer back to sabotaging thoughts. At the end of each day of this program, you'll create Response Cards to help carry out that day's task.

If your doctor gave you an antibiotic
to get rid of a bad infection, *would you take only
half the pill?* Of course not. Likewise, don't try
to take shortcuts with this program.

As time goes on, you'll have lots of sabotaging thoughts, but if you've been reading all your Response Cards regularly, you'll be ready to counteract them. The dieters I counsel tell me over and over again that these cards make a big difference for them. The cards prepare them to overcome their sabotaging thoughts, change their mindset, and do what they have to do to lose weight. It works for them—and it'll work for you, too.

what are you thinking?

You might still be having sabotaging thoughts about creating or reading your Advantages Response Card. If so, these responses may help.

Sabotaging Thought: I don't need to remind myself of the reasons to lose weight. I know them.
Helpful Response: I know them—now. But think about all the times I strayed from a diet in the past. I sure wasn't thinking of all the advantages of sticking to it then!

Sabotaging Thought: I don't feel like going to the trouble of getting index cards and writing down advantages right now. I'll do it later.
Helpful Response: To lose weight, I'm going to have to train myself to do what I need to do, not what I feel like doing at the moment. If I put off this task, I might end up never doing it.

Sabotaging Thought: This is too much effort.
Helpful Response: How much effort is it really? What's the big deal, anyway?

Sabotaging Thought: This won't work for me.
Helpful Response: I don't have a crystal ball, so I don't know whether or not it'll work. The one thing I do know for sure is that I didn't do this in the past and I haven't achieved lasting weight loss yet. I may as well just do it. What do I have to lose?

commit in writing

I'll read my Advantages Response Card at the following times: _____

_____
_____
_____
_____
_____
_____ .

My reminder system will be: _____

_____
_____
_____
_____
_____ .

Once I continually remind myself
of all the reasons I want to lose weight,
dieting will be easier.

today's to-do list

Check off the tasks you've completed. For any item you haven't completed, record when you're going to complete it.

_____ I created my Advantages Response Card.

_____ I wrote, recorded, or posted these advantages elsewhere.

_____ I implemented a reminder system.

day 2
Pick Two Reasonable Diets

I f you already know which diet you plan to follow, that's great. But keep reading because you need to choose *two* diets—the one you plan to start with and a second diet in case the first one doesn't work out.

The specific primary diet you choose doesn't matter, as long as it's healthy and well-balanced. You can choose a diet from a book, a Web site, a national health organization (such as one that promotes a diet that is healthy for your heart), a hospital or weight-loss clinic, or a commercial organization.

Before you pick this primary diet, though, you need to know that there are no miracle diets and that no one diet works equally well for all dieters. Although many diets are marketed as a "breakthrough" and "the easy way to lose weight," scientific research has determined that such sweeping claims are simply not true. *All* diets enable weight loss in the same way—by getting you to eat fewer calories.

It doesn't matter whether a diet directs you to consume certain combinations of food; to eat prescribed meals; or to count calories, grams, or predetermined numbers assigned to foods. The bottom line is that you'll still be taking in a limited number of calories. Researchers at the U.S. Department of Agriculture have determined that most people who don't vigorously exercise need to pare down their daily consumption to between 1,400 and 1,500 calories to lose weight. In fact, in a review of popular diets published in the journal *Obesity Research,* researchers found that the daily meal plans of several current popular diets each contain roughly 1,500 calories.

> *All diets enable weight loss
> in the same way*—by getting you
> to eat fewer calories.

Two Kinds of Diets

There are two basic types of diets: One type encourages you to follow a *set eating plan,* which provides a detailed prescription for meals and snacks. The other type is a *counting system,* which allows you to design your own meals and snacks—as long as you stay within a certain number of calories, carbohydrates, or assigned numbers.

There are pros and cons to both types.

Set Eating Plans

Pros: You don't have many choices. For some people, having a lack of choices is easier to deal with, especially initially. You can just tell yourself, *No candy at all,* and abide by this rule. Because you know what you're going to eat every day, you don't need to expend much mental energy on finding recipes or choosing foods.

Cons: This inflexibility can create a mindset of "good" foods and "bad" foods. If you slip and eat a bad food or something not on the meal plan, you might think that you've blown your diet and, therefore, might as well keep eating bad food for the rest of the day and start your diet again tomorrow. Another disadvantage is that you might not be able to sustain a set eating plan for the long term. Plus, with little or no flexibility, this type of plan doesn't allow for uncontrollable food circumstances, such as eating out or going on vacation.

Do you function better if you
have set rules to follow?
Or do you do better with more flexibility?

Counting Systems

Pros: You can more easily match your diet to your lifestyle, designing meals that work for you whenever you travel, eat out, or attend social gatherings. You can also ensure that your meals and snacks include all of your favorite foods.

Cons: These plans might provide you with *too* much flexibility. You can choose foods that aren't particularly healthy but still meet the set requirements. This type also takes more time and energy than a set eating plan to figure out what you're going to eat.

These are very broad definitions, as some diets contain elements of both types of plans. Think about diets that you've been on in the past. How well did any of these work for you? When choosing your diets (primary and back-up), think about what type of person you are: Do you function better if you have set rules to follow? Do you experience fewer cravings if you know that certain foods are completely off-limits on your diet? If so, then a set eating plan might work best for you. On the other hand, if you do better when you have more flexibility, then a counting system that guides your choices might work better.

Choose a diet that allows you to eat a reasonable variety of foods. *You might be able to lose weight on a diet that isn't nutritious, but eventually your body will rebel*—and you'll start to gain back weight.

Guidelines for a Doable Diet

In my experience, many dieters choose eating plans based on how quickly they expect the diet to help them lose weight. But rapid-weight-loss diets usually require you to eat fewer than 1,200 calories a day, and you'll have to endure more intense hunger than you would if you were following a diet that lets you eat more normally.

These types of deprivation diets can also backfire. They can negatively impact your energy level and mood. They also can slow your metabolism, which means the rate at which you lose weight starts to slow. Also, research shows that the large initial weight loss from these diets generally comes from the loss of body fluids, not from fat.

Even if you lose all of the weight you want on an extremely low-calorie diet, you're unlikely to be able to continue following such a plan over the long term. Research shows that nearly everyone who loses weight in this way quickly regains it.

Rather than basing your diet selection on speed, consider these factors:

Your diet should be healthy. Because you'll be following this diet for a long time, you need to select one that promotes good health. Choose a diet that allows you to eat a reasonable variety of foods. Be wary of any diet that unduly restricts healthy food choices. You might be able to lose weight on a diet that isn't nutritious, but eventually your body will rebel—and you'll start to gain back the excess weight.

tip! Show the diet you plan to follow to a nutritionist or to your health-care provider to make sure it's nutritionally sound and appropriate for you.

Choose a diet that includes food you like and can easily prepare. You'll be much more likely to stick to a diet that allows food you find both tasty and convenient. If you like the food, you'll more easily find the resolve to make the required recipes and to eat the required meals.

The Beck Diet Solution teaches you
how to *modify your diet by working planned
indulgences into your overall plan.* This can
help you stick to your diet long term.

Choose a diet that's flexible. You'll need to follow your diet in many different situations, such as dining out, vacations, business dinners, travel, and special occasions. Your meal plan must allow for these common life events—otherwise, you may find yourself backsliding.

Choose a diet that allows you to budget for indulgences. A diet that puts your favorite foods completely off-limits will likely lead you to crave those foods sooner or later. Even with a set eating plan, I've found that most people do better if they formulate a rule about what they can and what they *usually* can't eat, meaning they can periodically plan—in advance—to have small portions of "can't eat" foods.

For example, some dieters save 100 to 200 calories each day so that they can eat whatever they want in the evening after dinner. Other dieters or maintainers prefer to reserve one meal a week to eat certain foods not generally allowed on their diet plan.

The Beck Diet Solution teaches you how to eliminate spur-of-the-moment eating. I encourage you, however, to modify your diet by working *planned* indulgences into your overall plan. This can help you stick to your diet long term.

Learn from your past. Think about previous diets you've tried. Did you lose weight? Were the diets healthy, appetizing, and relatively convenient to follow? Perhaps there is a healthy diet you liked that worked fairly well. You might consider trying it again.

skipping meals

Are you tempted to speed weight loss by eating as little as possible or by skipping meals? Don't do it! Several studies have linked skipping meals, particularly breakfast, with weight *gain* rather than weight *loss*. If you skip a meal, you'll probably compensate for it later on. For example, research shows that people who habitually skip breakfast tend to seriously overeat at night. You might be better off, in fact, if you plan to eat up to six small meals a day.

Pick Your Diets Now

Before moving on to the next step in this plan, I want you to pick the primary diet you plan to follow, along with a backup diet. I've found that some dieters have to go through a process of trial and error before they find a diet they can follow for an extended period of time. You might find after a couple of weeks or months that the first diet you selected isn't working for you: You don't enjoy the suggested recipes, the meals are too complicated to prepare, or you really want foods not allowed by the diet. In that case, you can move on to Plan B.

Why pick a second diet now? If you become discouraged with your first diet, you'll be at risk for abandoning your weight-loss efforts altogether. If you know from the start what your fallback diet will be, you'll be much more likely to switch to it and to continue dieting without interruption.

To pick your diets, you can tap the following sources:

- Ask a health-care professional for suggestions.
- Consult with people you know who have lost weight.
- Talk to friends and family—those who know you well—about what kinds of diets they think will work for you.
- Go to the bookstore or library and look through diet books.
- Investigate commercial weight-loss programs.
- Look into nonprofit weight-loss group programs.
- Go online to investigate reputable Internet-based diets.
- Ask a nutritionist to develop a diet specific to your lifestyle and health needs.
- Join a weight-loss program at a local gym, hospital, or community center.

what are you thinking?

What's been going through your mind? When I told you about the importance of slow and steady weight loss, did you have any sabotaging thoughts? For example, did you find yourself thinking (as many dieters have revealed to me), *I have to lose 15 pounds in a month for a wedding [or some other special occasion] ... I have to go on a crash diet!*

If so, take the time right now to counter that type of thinking. For example, if you want to lose weight quickly for a special event, be realistic. Tell yourself that you're better off if you diet sensibly and lose just a little weight before the occasion and then continue to steadily lose weight afterwards.

Here are some other common sabotaging thoughts that I've heard over the years, along with helpful responses. Make Response Cards for any you think may apply to you.

Sabotaging Thought: I want to try this diet I heard about. It promises I can lose a lot of weight very quickly, very easily, and without effort. So what if it isn't nutritionally balanced? I won't be on it for long anyway.
Helpful Response: A fad diet isn't healthy, and I'll need to be on a diet—or a variation of the diet—for a long time. Promises that sound too good to be true invariably *are* too good to be true.

Sabotaging Thought: Since my diet doesn't say I have to eat breakfast, I'm going to skip it. I'd rather be able to eat more later in the day.
Helpful Response: Skipping breakfast in the past hasn't allowed me to lose weight permanently. I need to change my eating habits if I want to be successful this time.

Sabotaging Thought: I can learn to eat sensibly after I finish dieting.
Helpful Response: If I don't learn how to eat sensibly now, what evidence do I have that I'll be able to learn later? I need to start *now*.

Sabotaging Thought: I can lose weight only if I find exactly the right diet.
Helpful Response: There is no one right diet. There's nothing magical about any diet. The only formula for losing weight is taking in fewer calories than your body expends.

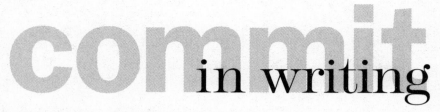

commit in writing

I picked a primary diet and a backup diet that are: _____
_____
_____.

(I hope you included "reasonable" and "nutritious.")

Once I accept the fact that
I have to follow a healthy eating plan
for life, dieting will be easier.

today's to-do list

Check off the tasks you've completed. For any item you haven't completed, record when you're going to complete it.

_____ I read my Advantages Response Card at least twice.

_____ I read other Response Cards as needed.

_____ I investigated diets.

_____ I chose a reasonable primary diet and a backup diet.

day 3
Eat Sitting Down

If you always eat sitting down, you've already mastered this important step. However, if you've struggled with your weight and dieted on and off for many years, my guess is that you probably do some eating while standing. You also probably have a tendency to rationalize or perhaps not even notice how much you've eaten. Opportunities to eat while standing up abound.

Do you do any of the following?

- Take free samples of food at the grocery store.
- Taste food as you prepare meals.
- Sneak bits of food from someone's plate as you clear the table.
- Spoon ice cream out of the container or reach into a bag of chips while you're walking around talking on the phone.
- Take a piece of candy or a pretzel as you walk past the snack jar sitting on a coworker's desk.
- Nibble on something you see when opening the refrigerator to get something else out.

When you think about it now, I'm sure you recognize that all calories add up. But at the moment you're actually eating, you might rationalize what you're doing with the sabotaging thought, *It won't really matter if I eat this.*

Today, you'll make a commitment to sit down every single time you eat something—even if it's just a bite. Are you thinking, *Why do I have to do this? What's the big deal about eating while I'm standing up?* Well, here's why you have to adopt a strict rule about sitting down to eat:

You absolutely need to become more conscious of everything you put in your mouth. You need to pay full attention to what you're eating so you don't say to yourself, *I'm still hungry ... I want more,* when you've finished your allotted food.

Most of the eating that people do while on their feet is *impulse* eating, not food that they had planned to eat. When you sit down to eat, especially at

I'm sure you recognize that *all calories add up.* But at the moment you're actually eating, you might rationalize what you're doing.

your dining table, you've made a *conscious* decision to eat. You know these calories count, and you can more easily monitor what you eat—and, thus, avoid overeating. In essence, you're telling yourself, *I'm sitting down, having a proper meal (or snack), and I'm eating what I'm supposed to be eating.* When you impulsively eat standing up, you're telling yourself that it's okay to give in to this urge to eat, that it doesn't really matter, and that there won't be any consequences. But there *will* be consequences because *every bite of food you put in your mouth has calories.* Even if you're only eating raw carrots while you're standing up today, you might be eating chocolate while you're standing up tomorrow.

You'll feel more satisfied. Since you'll be eating less food, it's important to see all of it spread in front of you at meal or snack time so you can be more visually satisfied. The less food you see, the more deprived you'll feel.

Let's say you're having cereal and an orange for breakfast. If you eat the cereal standing up, you'll probably eat it too quickly or absentmindedly. And then when you sit down, you'll have only the orange left, and you probably won't feel satisfied.

Here's another example: You're at a warehouse grocery store and try several of the free samples of food, which you eat while you're wandering around. Now you go home for dinner. You can eat only half of what your diet prescribes because of the calories you consumed at the store.

> Since you'll be eating less food,
> *it's important for you to see all of it spread
> in front of you at meal or snack time*
> so you can be more visually satisfied.

When you eat standing up, you might feel physically as full as if you had eaten sitting down, *but you won't feel as psychologically satisfied.* Tasting, chewing, and swallowing food gives you a certain degree of satisfaction, but you also need visual satisfaction. You have to make the most of every bite.

Many of the dieters I've counseled have told me that learning to eat only when seated was key to their success at losing weight and maintaining the loss. It was crucial to my own success—it also was one of the hardest skills to incorporate into my life. I had a tough time with it in the beginning, but now I eat *almost* everything sitting down, except for a few raw vegetables that I plan to eat while I prepare dinner. (No one's perfect!) Every time I slip back into the habit of eating standing up, I invariably gain weight.

How to Sit Consistently

Stop yourself whenever you're tempted to eat while standing. Remind yourself why it's important: Even if you can get away *now* with eating while standing, you're putting yourself at risk for gaining weight at some point in the future. You have to make eating while sitting a lifelong habit.

So make it your goal to sit down whenever you eat. Consider placing a note that says "Sit down" in your appointment book, diet notebook, or on your refrigerator or cabinet door. It might also help to reset the table immediately after finishing a snack or meal as a reminder to sit down the next time you eat.

what are you thinking?

You might find that the urge to eat while standing persists and that sabotaging thoughts get in your way. Be prepared to write Response Cards. Here are some common sabotaging thoughts with suggested responses.

Sabotaging Thought: I enjoy spontaneous munching. I don't want to stop eating while I'm standing.
Helpful Response: I need to sit down to eat. When I eat standing up, I just don't notice what I'm eating. I could eat way too much without realizing it. If I want to be thinner, I have to impose this rule on myself. I might not want to give up this behavior, but I'll enjoy being thinner so much more.

Sabotaging Thought: It's okay if I eat standing up this one time. I'll eat my next meal sitting down.
Helpful Response: "Just this one time" is not okay. I have to face the fact that I probably can't lose weight or keep it off if I refuse to change my habit of eating while standing up.

Sabotaging Thought: I don't have time to sit down to eat.
Helpful Response: Sitting down isn't optional. I'll have to rearrange my schedule so that I *do* have time. It's essential for controlling what and how much I eat.

commit in writing

When I feel like eating standing up, I'm going to: _____
_____
_____
_____
_____.

I'm going to remind myself to sit down when I eat by: _____
_____
_____
_____
_____.

Once I accept the fact that
I have to eat everything sitting down,
dieting will be easier.

today's to-do list

Check off the tasks you've completed. For any item you haven't completed, record when you're going to complete it.

_____ I read my Advantages Response Card at least twice.

_____ I read other Response Cards as needed.

_____ I created a Response Card to encourage myself to sit while eating.

_____ I created a reminder system so I'll remember to sit while eating.

_____ I sat down when I ate.

Circle one: Every time   Most of the time   Some of the time

day 4
Give Yourself Credit

I've noticed that people who struggle with their weight tend to be hard on themselves. The moment they stray, they become self-critical. Instead of viewing slips as mistakes and thinking how they can solve the problem the next time it arises, they tell themselves that they're weak, hopeless, or even bad.

Do you have a tendency to focus on the negative, berating yourself for everything you do wrong? To counteract this tendency, it's important for you to learn to give yourself credit for everything you do *right*.

Start now by telling yourself, *Good job,* or the equivalent every time you sit down to eat, read a Response Card, and complete every other weight-loss task in this program. By consciously giving yourself credit, you'll reinforce your self-confidence and build an awareness that you're strong and in control. When you overeat or eat in an unplanned way, you might begin to feel helpless, thinking, *I just can't make myself do what I need to do.* When you give yourself credit every time you do something right, though, you can more easily see such slips as momentary mistakes, not earthshaking events, and head off a sense of hopelessness.

tip!

Create a "credit account." For every positive behavior you acknowledge, drop a coin or dollar bill (whatever is handy) into a special container. After you follow your diet plan for a certain number of weeks (you decide how many), take the money out, add whatever extra amount is required, and buy something for yourself that you might normally pass up, such as tickets to a play or sporting event.

How and When to Give Yourself Credit

Giving yourself credit can take the form of a word or brief phrase that you say silently to yourself, such as:

- *Okay!*
- *That was good.*
- *Great!*
- *Good going!*
- *That deserves credit.*
- *Yes!*
- *I did it!*

it's all in your mind

Giving yourself credit just takes a moment, but it's *essential* in your weight-loss efforts. To understand the importance of giving credit, consider these scenarios:

Scenario 1

Sue is at a restaurant for a large family reunion. She sees bread—which is many dieters' downfall—on the table as soon as she sits down, but tells herself, *I'm not going to eat it ... I can wait for my meal to come.* She tries to resist the bread, but her dining companions each take a slice, remark how delicious it tastes, and keep passing the basket. Finally, she reaches in for a piece and eats it. Then she tells herself, *I can't believe I was so weak ... I have no willpower whatsoever.* She gives up, proceeds to eat another slice, and then overeats for the rest of the evening.

Scenario 2

Peter is at the same restaurant. He, too, is tempted by the smell of the bread. His mouth starts to water, especially when he sees his friend eating the bread with gusto. After resisting for a while, he finally eats a slice. He then tells himself, *Okay, so I gave in ... At least I resisted the breadbasket for 10 minutes ... I deserve credit for that ... The last time I tried to diet, I couldn't make myself wait at all ... And it's good I've eaten only one slice ... I'll make sure to eat just a quarter of the baked potato I ordered, instead of half.* Peter gets right back on track and stays within his calorie limit for the day.

In the first scenario, Sue's self-critical thinking eroded her confidence, leading her to eat even more bread. In the second scenario, giving himself at least partial credit allowed Peter to regroup, start fresh, and stay within his diet.

Start giving yourself credit today and continue to give yourself credit whenever you engage in a helpful eating behavior. For example, look at what you've achieved after just three days on this program. You deserve credit for:

- Creating and reading your Advantages Response Card
- Creating and reading other Response Cards
- Investigating and choosing a primary diet and a backup diet
- Sitting while eating
- Recognizing and answering back your sabotaging thoughts
- Filling out the to-do list at the end of each day
- Reading—and rereading—this book

You also deserve credit every time you refrain from engaging in unhelpful behaviors. When you've finished eating, look for ways to give yourself credit for refraining from doing the unhelpful things you're tempted to do, such as the following:

- Wanting to eat walking around, standing, or lounging, but not doing so
- Refraining from taking second helpings
- Refusing a free sample at the grocery store
- Ignoring the baked goods someone brought to work

Giving myself credit is a skill I had to learn—but now it comes easily to me. I give myself credit throughout the day, whenever I finish a task or even part of a task. I say to myself, *Good, that's done,* even if it's just writing two more paragraphs of an article or brushing my teeth. It's quite easy for me to give myself credit when I eat right: *Good, I ate what I'd planned.* It's now especially easy for me to give myself credit when I pass up food I hadn't planned to eat, as I did this morning at a breakfast buffet: *Good, I'm glad I didn't eat a doughnut, a bagel, and a lot of other stuff.*

As you practice this skill, giving yourself credit will become more and more automatic (as it has for me). Right now, however, you might need a system to help you remember to recognize your positive behaviors. Here are some suggestions to help you get started:

Write down the word *credit* on a sticky note. Place it on your refrigerator, in your appointment book, on the dashboard of your car, or in other places where you'll often see it. Consider turning it into a screen saver for your computer.

tip!

If you find you're self-critical every time you make a mistake in your eating, you'll undermine your confidence. If you eat something you hadn't planned to eat or if you mindlessly eat standing up, for example, beware of overly harsh sabotaging thoughts. Make sure you tell yourself something similar to the following: *This is hard. I'll get better at it. Next time, I can....*

Whenever you see this word, ask yourself, *Which positive things did I do (or what unhelpful things did I refrain from doing) today?*

Once or twice a day, pull out your diet notebook. Think about the past few hours and make a list of credit-worthy behaviors.

Every time you check off an item on your daily to-do list, say something positive to yourself. In fact, instead of making a check mark, you might want to draw a star or a plus sign.

Reflect on your eating behaviors whenever you finish a meal or snack. Ask yourself, *Did I remember to eat slowly? Did I notice every bite? Did I stop when the food was gone and refrain from taking seconds?*

Buy a small counter—the kind that people use to keep track of how much their groceries cost while they're shopping or that golfers use to keep track of their score—and click it every time you deserve credit. At the end of the day, record the number of clicks in your diet notebook.

what are you thinking?

Are you having any sabotaging thoughts about giving yourself credit? Here are some typical ones, along with helpful responses. Create Response Cards for any you think apply to you.

Sabotaging Thought: I don't deserve credit for doing things I should already be doing. These things aren't accomplishments. They should be easy for me to do.
Helpful Response: If I don't give myself credit for essential behaviors, I'll be less likely to practice these behaviors consistently. If I were naturally thin, had a small appetite, and didn't have to work at controlling my weight, perhaps I wouldn't deserve credit. But I'm *not* naturally thin. I *do* struggle. I *do* deserve credit every single time I think about something in a helpful way or engage in helpful behavior.

Sabotaging Thought: It feels unnatural to give myself credit.
Helpful Response: Giving myself credit is a skill that I'll build over time. It's okay if it seems forced in the beginning. The more I practice this skill, the better I'll get at it and the more automatic and natural it will become.

Sabotaging Thought: It feels too juvenile to praise myself.
Helpful Response: It's not foolish to praise myself; it's absolutely essential to building my confidence. I'll need confidence to get through the harder times.

Sabotaging Thought: I don't deserve credit until I've lost all the weight that I want to lose.
Helpful Response: It's counterproductive to wait. I need to strengthen the part of my mind that believes I can follow the program. I'm only human and might stray from my plan from time to time. When this happens, a sense of helplessness might kick in. Continually building my confidence by giving myself credit can protect me from feeling helpless and hopeless and from throwing in the towel. And, actually, the process of losing weight is the hardest part. Once I've learned the skills I need, maintaining my weight will be easier. So I deserve lots of credit now, while I'm working the hardest.

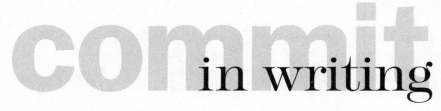

commit in writing

To remember to give myself credit consistently, I'm going to: _____
_____
_____
_____.

> Once I build my confidence by giving
> myself credit, dieting will be easier.

today's to-do list

Check off the tasks you've completed. For any item you haven't completed, record when you're going to complete it.

_____ I read my Advantages Response Card at least twice today.

_____ I read other Response Cards as needed.

_____ I created a reminder system for giving myself credit.

_____ I sat down to eat.

      Circle one: Every time   Most of the time   Some of the time

_____ I gave myself credit for sitting down to eat.

      Circle one: Every time   Most of the time   Some of the time

day 5
Eat Slowly and Mindfully

There are two very beneficial reasons that it's important to always eat slowly and to pay particular attention to what you're eating:

- When you eat slowly, your brain has time to register that you're full.
- When you notice and enjoy every mouthful, you feel more satisfied when the food is gone.

From talking to dieters, there's no question in my mind that eating too quickly and mindlessly is common among people who have a weight problem. How quickly do you eat? Do you sometimes feel deprived when you're finished eating? Have you had the experience of eating a reasonably sized meal and then saying to yourself, *That wasn't much food at all ... I'm still hungry,* because you hadn't paid enough attention to the food you ate?

Research shows that there's a lag—up to 20 minutes—between when your stomach fills up and when your brain gets the message that you're full. The more slowly you eat, the more time you give the "I'm full" alert to reach your brain so that it can signal you to stop eating.

eat slowly

Studies show that people do indeed eat less when they eat slowly. In one study conducted at Louisiana State University in Baton Rouge, researchers gave a group of overweight individuals a lunch of chicken nuggets and timed their eating pace. Then the researchers fed the same volunteers a series of lunches over a period of days, instructing them to take bites only when they heard a computer beep. Participants were allowed to stop eating whenever they felt full.

The researchers varied the pace of eating during each meal. For one meal, the computer beeped about twice as slowly as the participants' normal eating pace. For another, the computer beeped at the participants' usual faster eating pace. For a third lunch, the computer beeped faster for part of the meal and more slowly at the end of the meal.

The results? All of the participants ended up eating less whenever the computer beeped more slowly.

How to Slow Down

If you habitually eat quickly, switching to a slower eating pace might feel unnatural at first. You might need to remind yourself to put down your utensils several times during the meal and to wait 10 to 30 seconds before picking them up again. Practice the following strategies until you naturally eat more slowly.

Change something in your eating environment. For example, use a cloth napkin instead of a paper one. Use different dishes (or paper plates) or a new place mat. Change the flatware you usually use. Put a vase or another object directly in front of your plate. Every time you notice something different on the table, remind yourself, *Oh, yes, this means I'm supposed to eat slowly.*

Set a timer to beep every one to three minutes. If changing something in your environment isn't compelling enough, perhaps the timer will help. Each time you hear a beep, put down your flatware. Wait at least 10 seconds and, when you pick up your utensils again, remind yourself to eat slowly.

Take sips of water after every few bites. While water doesn't offer any magical weight-loss power, drinking between mouthfuls of food does slow down your eating.

Eat something hot. Starting your meal with soup (if it's allowed on your food plan), for example, forces you to eat slowly and to practice this skill.

Pay attention to your body. Look for signs that you're starting to feel full. Becoming conscious of how your body feels can remind you to slow down.

Look at the clock. Notice what time it is at the beginning and at the end of your meal. In your diet notebook or on a sticky note that you can keep on your refrigerator, write down how long it takes you to eat. At each meal, try to slow down and draw it out just a bit longer.

How to Notice What You're Eating

It's very easy to become distracted when you eat, which can reduce the degree of satisfaction you're getting from your food. Here are some tips to help you concentrate:

Eat in a relaxed atmosphere. The less stress you feel, the more easily you'll be able to pay attention to what you're eating. Do what you can to eat in a quiet, nonstimulating environment.

Focus intently on your food. Savor the taste of each bite, noting the flavor and texture of everything you eat.

Train yourself to eat with some distractions. It's best to minimize distractions

solve problems

It can be difficult to eat slowly and mindfully when you have a lot of responsibilities to fulfill. Here are suggestions for some specific difficulties (ask a friend for help with other problems).

The Kids. There are lots of nice things about family life, but eating in a relaxing atmosphere is often not one of them. It's easy to lose track of what you're eating and how you're eating when you have to pay attention to small children. Some of the dieters I work with alternate supervision with their spouses or partners. You might want to try this strategy, too.

For example, once everyone is seated at the table, you eat just part of your meal, as slowly and mindfully as you can. When the kids leave the table, you get up, too. Supervise the kids for 10 to 15 minutes while your spouse finishes eating and then switch so your spouse can do the supervision while you finish your meal. (Thank goodness for microwaves, so you can reheat your food.) The next night, do it the opposite way.

Breakfast Time. If you're too rushed in the mornings, you can do a different sort of switch. Move as many morning tasks as possible to the evening. Maybe you can shower, lay out your clothes, pack your lunch, and then straighten up the house before you go to sleep. Also, get out of bed earlier, if necessary. Make eating a proper breakfast slowly and mindfully a real priority, so that you can achieve your goal of losing weight.

It's best to minimize distractions when you eat, but ultimately you'll need to learn the skill of eating mindfully even if you're distracted.

when you eat by refraining from reading, watching TV, or using the computer. While this is a desirable goal, I've found most people just won't do this long term. Even if you aren't engaging in one of these activities, you're bound to get distracted if you eat with other people and carry on a conversation.

Try eating without distractions for just a few meals until you really master the skills of eating slowly and fully noticing what you eat. Then incorporate these skills into your normal eating conditions. Whenever you find that you've eaten too quickly or mindlessly, try to eat the next meal without distractions to sharpen your skills.

what are you thinking?

Do you have any sabotaging thoughts about this step in the program? If so, make Response Cards based on the relevant thoughts and responses below.

Sabotaging Thought: If I don't eat quickly, I'll inconvenience: _____

_____ .

Helpful Response: It isn't reasonable for me to sacrifice my needs. I deserve to enjoy what I'm eating. I deserve to engage in healthy behaviors to reach my goals.

Sabotaging Thought: I'm a fast eater. That's just the way I am.
Helpful Response: Being a fast eater probably contributed to my weight gain. I can't have it both ways. I can't eat quickly and also lose weight and maintain my weight loss. Even though eating more slowly will take effort and feel unnatural in the beginning, I'll get used to it and then I won't have to think much about it.

Sabotaging Thought: I truly don't have time to eat slowly.
Helpful Response: I need to rearrange my schedule to *make* the time. If I needed to take time for a lifesaving medical procedure three times a day, I'd somehow find the time. I'm not giving eating properly a high enough priority.

commit in writing

When I feel like eating quickly, I'm going to: _____

_____

_____

_____

_____

_____.

To remind myself to eat slowly, I'm going to: _____

_____

_____

_____

_____.

Once I accept the fact that I have
to eat slowly and notice every bite,
dieting will be easier.

today's to-do list

Check off the tasks you've completed. For any item you haven't completed, record when you're going to complete it.

_____ I read my Advantages Response Card at least twice.

_____ I read other Response Cards as needed.

_____ I ate slowly, sitting down and noticing every bite.

Circle one: Every time   Most of the time   Some of the time

_____ I gave myself credit when I engaged in helpful dieting behaviors.

Circle one: Every time   Most of the time   Some of the time

day 6

Find a Diet Coach

Yes, you're going to need a diet coach. Are you having any sabotaging thoughts? Perhaps you prefer to keep your diet private. Or maybe you're uncomfortable with asking for help. In my experience, however, very few people who have struggled with dieting can lose weight and sustain that weight loss without help and encouragement from another person. Studies consistently show that getting someone to support you increases your chance of success.

In many ways, I'm serving as your diet coach. Through the pages of this book, I'm providing you with the same advice that I've given to dieters over the years. But you also need a real live person to talk to, someone you like and on whom you can depend. Here's what your diet coach can do:

Keep you motivated. Your diet coach can encourage you by helping you remember why all of your efforts are worthwhile. Give him or her a copy of your Advantages Response Card. When you're on the verge of giving into a craving—when those sabotaging thoughts pop up—turn to your coach. If you start getting discouraged and want to throw in the towel, your coach (as keeper of your memories) can remind you that you don't usually feel that way and that most of the time you actually feel good about dieting.

Build your self-confidence. Your diet coach can help make sure that you give yourself credit on an ongoing basis. And when you slip and think, *I can't do this anymore,* your diet coach can help you get back on track and remind you of what you've learned to get to that point. Your diet coach can counteract your sense of helplessness.

Help you solve problems. From time to time, you'll encounter obstacles that can make sticking to this program difficult. You might discover that you're too busy to find the time and energy you need to follow your diet. You might feel unmotivated. You might find that other people, purposely or not, put roadblocks in your way. Let your diet coach help you solve both your diet- and non-diet-related problems. Two heads are better than one!

Few people who have struggled with dieting *can lose weight* and sustain that weight loss *without help and encouragement from another person.*

Keep you accountable. Knowing that you have to report on your progress to someone can motivate you to stick to your plan. THIS IS A CRUCIAL COMPONENT OF THE PROGRAM. Dieters I've counseled have told me time and time again, "I didn't overeat because I knew I'd have to tell you about it." You'll keep yourself in line better if you know you're going to have to report to your diet coach. Make sure you're completely honest!

> Knowing that *you have to report on your progress to someone else* can motivate you to stick to your plan.

Help you take a more useful perspective. Imagine your diet coach looking over your shoulder at times when your resolve is weak. When you consider straying from your food plan, think to yourself, *What would my coach say to me now?* Doing so can help you better stick to your plan.

How to Find a Diet Coach

Decide whom you'd like to be your diet coach and line up that person now. You might not need your coach's help at this point to assist you in implementing the tasks in the program. And you might not need the inspiration your coach can provide during the first few weeks

tip! Whenever your diet coach says something helpful, record it in your diet notebook so you'll be able to refer to it in the future.

of dieting, when your motivation is high. But you *will* need a diet coach at some point. Lining up your diet coach now is important because I've found that a dieter is much less likely to try to find a coach once he or she has hit a rough patch and is feeling discouraged—which is the time, of course, when the coach is needed most. If you're not sure whom to select, consider doing the following:

Enlist the help of a close friend or family member. It isn't necessary to select someone who has had experience with dieting. It's more important to choose someone who is positive; good at problem solving; and truly supportive, motivating, and proud of you.

Consider starting this program with a friend or family member. Some dieters find it very helpful to choose someone who also wants to lose weight, so that they can be each other's diet coach.

You want a diet coach who helps you identify and counter your unhelpful thinking, gives practical advice, is highly encouraging and motivating, and is willing to help you implement this program.

Join an organized group. Look into weight-loss support groups offered by nonprofit community groups, hospitals, and commercial organizations. Ask to sit in on a meeting before making a commitment. You don't want a group in which people just talk about their problems and express their negative emotions in a nonconstructive way. You want a group in which people describe their successes, help others with their diet-related difficulties, and share useful weight-loss strategies.

If you join a group, you won't feel alone, since you're sharing experiences with others who are also struggling. Viewing their slips and mistakes in an objective, problem-solving way can help you take a more useful view of your own difficulties. You might also get a good feeling from helping others—and from being helped by them. You might meet someone who will agree to be your diet coach—and vice versa!

Find a diet professional. Consider working one-on-one with a mental-health or health-care professional who has had experience and success with helping people lose weight and keep it off. You don't want to pick someone who focuses only on the supposed root cause of your weight problems ("It's your mother's fault!"). You want someone who helps you identify and counter your unhelpful thinking, gives practical advice, is highly encouraging and motivating, and is willing to help you implement this program.

Investigate Internet support. Face-to-face interaction is usually more desirable, but if you absolutely can't meet with someone in person, investigate weight-loss support groups on the Internet. A study conducted at the University of Vermont in Burlington found that participants who enrolled in a weight-maintenance program over the Internet sustained the same amount of weight loss as participants who met with a support group in person.

What to Discuss with Your Coach

Your coach can help you in many ways. Ideally, schedule a regular time to talk (face-to-face, if possible), at least once a week and then in between by phone or by e-mail on an as-needed basis—daily, if necessary.

During your scheduled weekly meetings, you should talk about:

- Your change in weight during the past week. You don't have to state your actual weight, just how much the scale went up or down.
- The successes you had during the past week. Use the to-do lists at the end of each day to report on what you've done. Mention anything else that you deserve credit for, so your diet coach can positively reinforce what you've done.
- The struggles you had in the past week. Talk about your cravings, slipups, or life stressors. Mention anything that might interfere with executing the steps of this program. Ask your coach to help you find ways to deal with setbacks and challenges in the future. Report your sabotaging thoughts and ask for help with how to respond to them.

Initiate communication at key times when:

- You're going into high-risk situations—such as a party or family celebration—in which you're concerned you might stray. Together, figure out which strategies you'll need to use.
- You've strayed from your plan. Discuss what you need to do now to get right back on track. You might especially need help if you're criticizing yourself and feeling like a failure.

Call or e-mail daily if:

- You're struggling to stick to your daily eating plan. I've found that some people need to give an account to their coach of what they ate during the day every evening for the first few weeks or longer. It's the only way they can stick to their eating plan. They've told me that they often didn't eat certain foods because they didn't want to have to report it.
- You're struggling to complete other daily tasks in this program. You won't have to depend on your diet coach forever. All your struggles will get easier and easier as time goes on.

Every evening for the first few weeks or longer, some people need to give an account of what they ate during the day.

what are you thinking?

Are you having sabotaging thoughts about lining up a diet coach? Check to see if any of these thoughts are familiar and use the helpful responses as guides to creating Response Cards for yourself.

Sabotaging Thought: What if I get a diet coach and then fail? He or she will think poorly of me.
Helpful Response: If I pick the right person, I'll maximize my chances of success. I'm not going to choose a diet coach who will view me negatively just for trying.

Sabotaging Thought: I don't want to impose on someone.
Helpful Response: First, whomever I select as my diet coach will probably consider me worth the trouble. Second, serving as my support person probably isn't as burdensome as I might believe. Third, the process might well bring us closer together. Many people feel honored to serve as support to someone else. Finally, I can at least give someone the choice of whether or not to help me.

Sabotaging Thought: I should be able to do this by myself.
Helpful Response: If I could do it by myself, I'd have already lost weight and kept it off. I need to face the fact that I need help—just as many other people do.

Sabotaging Thought: I strayed from my diet plan, and I think I gained weight. I don't want to call and tell my diet coach.
Helpful Response: This is the time I need my diet coach most. In a few minutes, I'll probably be glad I called. My diet coach won't criticize me or think poorly of me. If I call, I'll get the practical help and support I need. The reasons to lose weight that I wrote on my Advantages Response Card are still important to me, so I should go ahead and call now.

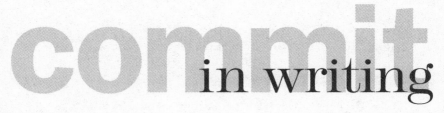

commit in writing

I'll ask _____ to be my diet coach.

Once I have a diet coach who is
regularly supporting me and helping
me, dieting will be easier.

today's to-do list

Check off the tasks you've completed. For any item you haven't completed, record when you're going to complete it.

_____ I read my Advantages Response Card at least twice today.

_____ I read other Response Cards as needed.

_____ I ate slowly, sitting down and noticing every bite.

Circle one: Every time   Most of the time   Some of the time

_____ I gave myself credit when I engaged in helpful dieting behaviors.

Circle one: Every time   Most of the time   Some of the time

_____ I decided on a diet coach or support group.

_____ I took steps to line up support.

day 7

Arrange Your Environment

I find it difficult to have junk food staring me in the face. At home, I make sure it's all on a high shelf in a cupboard or in the freezer. I don't keep food in my office or in my car because I don't always have the mental energy to resist urges to eat—particularly at the end of the workday. The dieters with whom I work also have found this practice to be a valuable strategy for losing weight and maintaining their weight loss.

It's especially important to avoid environmental triggers when you're first starting your diet. "Out of sight, out of mind" is a good policy right now. Although you won't necessarily have to reduce environmental triggers forever, you may decide, as I have, that you prefer to keep certain foods out of sight even after you've lost weight. Today, I'd like you to prepare your home and work environments by putting tempting foods where you won't easily see them—and by putting wholesome foods allowed by your diet in plain view.

Did this suggestion trigger sabotaging thoughts? Many dieters tell me, "If I make changes, I'll have to tell everyone I'm dieting. I'm worried I could fail on this diet, too. Then everyone will know. So it's better not to let anyone know." If you're having such thoughts, you're going to need a strong response or you may decide not to make environmental changes. Consider the following:

You don't have to tell people you're dieting. You can tell them that you've decided to eat in a more healthful way.

How differently will people really view you? No matter what happens, if they've had a positive view of you, they'll probably still think of you positively.

Won't most people think it's better to have tried to diet than not to have tried at all? They'll probably see your efforts at self-improvement as an admirable goal, even if all doesn't turn out as you expected or hoped.

Finally, think about how likely it is that you *will* lose weight this time—because now you have the power of Cognitive Therapy and the Beck Diet Solution—*if you follow all the steps.* Now, are you ready to read about how you need to change your environment?

Prepare your home and work environments by putting tempting foods where you won't easily see them—and by putting wholesome foods allowed by your diet in plain view.

Changes at Home

Follow these suggestions for reducing food triggers in your kitchen:

Remove your personal temptations. Open all of the food cabinets and, if at all possible, give away or throw out the foods that could tempt you to go off your diet plan. Don't worry about throwing out food. It's going to get wasted one way or another—either in the trash can or in your body. Or, second best, move these foods to the back of the shelf or to a high shelf. Do the same in your refrigerator and freezer.

Rearrange your dishes. Some people overeat when they use large dishes and utensils. Researchers at the University of Illinois at Urbana-Champaign found that partygoers who used large spoons or large bowls scooped considerably more ice cream than those who used smaller utensils and bowls. If you think it would help, reorganize your plates and bowls so that the smallest ones are easiest to reach.

Consider others. If you share your kitchen with others, you need to enlist their cooperation to keep tempting foods out of your sight. Although everyone in your household would probably benefit from junking the junk food, it might not be realistic for you to insist they do so. Here are some things you *can* do:

- Tell everyone at home that you're going to be eating in a more healthful way. You don't have to disclose that you're trying to lose weight unless you want to.
- Ask other adults for their help. Rather than demand that they also make changes, phrase your request like this, "Would you be willing to help me by...?"
- Announce to your children the changes you intend to make. Don't ask for their permission. You, not they, should be in charge of what goes on in the kitchen.
- If anyone resists the changes you want to make, say that you're open to other solutions. If you reach an impasse, consult your diet coach for additional ideas.

Do creative problem solving. The dieters I've worked with have come up with a number of strategies to reduce environmental triggers.

When Cindy started her diet, she made the following rule: *No candy in the house.* Once a week, however, she would take her kids to the store, and they could choose one serving of whatever candy they wanted as a treat.

Phillip asked his teenage kids to buy only a single-sized serving of certain foods (one small bag of corn chips, one small package of bite-sized doughnuts, one individual-sized pie) at a time.

Maria, a teenager, asked her parents to keep all of the junk food in a special box in the broom closet.

Meg had to be inventive. Her husband loved to eat potato chips and other snack foods. When she mentioned that she really wanted these foods out of the house, he wasn't willing to give them up. So they came to a compromise: He kept the snack foods in his car instead of in the kitchen. He also agreed to buy just one bagel at a time for himself and not keep extras in the freezer.

Changes at Work

Where do you find food at work? Do certain foods remain in plain sight in the office break room? Do some of your coworkers keep candy or other treats on their desks for others to enjoy? Is there a coffee shop or gift shop in your building that sells snacks? Are there vending machines in your lunchroom? Are baked goods served at meetings?

The easy availability of these foods is counterproductive to your good intentions. It can be hard to ask others at work to make changes, but it will be worth it. Provide a rationale and phrase your request as a question: "I'm trying to eat in a more healthful way. Would you be willing to...?"

Here are some strategies that have worked for the dieters I've counseled:

- Ask coworkers who keep candy or snack foods on their desks if they wouldn't mind moving their snack jars to a less-visible location. Or buy each of them an attractive opaque jar for their snacks as a special gift.
- Ask coworkers who leave food in the break room for others to share if they'd mind if you moved the food out of sight. Say that you'd be happy to leave a note in its place directing where to find it.
- Talk to your boss about starting a healthy eating campaign at work. See if you can arrange for raw vegetables or fruits to be served at meetings instead of (or in addition to) baked goods.
- Ask for more healthful foods in the cafeteria.
- Try to arrange for at least *some* healthier food selections in the vending machines.

Anna worked with people who frequently brought in cakes, doughnuts, cookies, and pastries to share with others in the office. She usually was able to resist eating these foods until the middle of the afternoon when she became tired and her resolve weakened. She didn't feel it was right to ask her coworkers not to bring in food, so she thought of a good solution. Anna approached one of her coworkers, explained her dilemma about the food, and offered a suggestion: Would the coworker mind if Anna moved her cupcakes from the counter to inside the cabinet? Anna offered to post a note reading: "Cupcakes inside, courtesy of Shelly." Shelly immediately agreed. Anna found it much easier to resist the baked goods once they were out of sight, even though she knew where to find them. She was pleasantly surprised when several people thanked her for moving them.

You need to be realistic; you won't be able to eliminate *all* environmental triggers at work. As time goes by, it'll become much easier for you to resist temptation. In the meantime, consider a compromise, such as taking a small portion of food and saving it for later, or eating a small portion at a time when you won't be tempted to eat more. The latter is a strategy that worked well for David, a dieter I counseled. He decided that he would choose one snack (whatever he wanted) from the vending machine once a week—even though it wasn't on his list of permitted foods. However, he allowed himself to buy this snack only on Fridays and just before quitting time. Although he had to pass the snack machine many times a day, he was able to resist buying treats at other times by reminding himself, *I'll have it on Friday.*

At the office where Donna worked, they served chocolate chip cookies every Tuesday afternoon during a meeting. She decided that she would wrap up one cookie each time, take it home, and eat it for her evening snack in place of the fruit that her eating plan recommended.

> *Consider a compromise,* such as taking a small portion of food and saving it for later or eating a small portion at a time when you won't be tempted to eat more.

what are you thinking?

If you have reservations about doing today's task, you're probably having sabotaging thoughts. Making environmental changes is important. Get out your index cards and prepare your responses. The following sample responses might be helpful.

Sabotaging Thought: If I make changes, I'll have to tell other people that I'm dieting.
Helpful Response: What's the big deal, really? The worst that can happen is that someone will be mildly critical of me if I don't lose weight. On the other hand, this program is probably exactly what I need to succeed this time. Announcing my intention to eat in a more healthful way (I don't have to say that I'm dieting) makes it more likely that others will go along with the changes I need to make. And it'll be such a relief not to feel tempted every time I walk into the kitchen or encounter food at work.

Sabotaging Thought: I shouldn't inconvenience other people.
Helpful Response: Whom will I inconvenience the most? How inconvenient will these environmental changes really be compared to how much benefit I'll get? And other people will likely benefit from the changes I make.

Sabotaging Thought: If I tell my family or coworkers about my diet, they'll make comments about what I eat.
Helpful Response: I can ask them not to say anything: "It would help if you didn't comment on what I eat or don't eat—can you do that for me?"

Sabotaging Thought: I shouldn't put my needs above the needs of my family.
Helpful Response: I'm entitled to work toward a goal that's important to me. It's time for me to practice meeting my needs. Besides, my family doesn't need junk food. They'd be better off if they didn't eat it either.

Sabotaging Thought: My family or coworkers will get mad at me for these changes.
Helpful Response: Am I thinking realistically? How mad could they get? How long will they stay mad? Is it reasonable for them to get mad? Remember, I'm not doing this to make them mad. I'm doing this because I need to.

Sabotaging Thought: I don't know if I really want to change my environment.
Helpful Response: Well, that may be true, but it's even more important to me to lose weight. I can't have it both ways. I can't resist making changes *and* lose weight. I'll go read my Advantages Response Card right now.

Sabotaging Thought: I don't want to waste food by throwing it out.
Helpful Response: If I don't throw it out, I'll be at risk for "wasting" it in my body, where it'll turn to fat. Which is a better way to waste it?

commit in writing

I'll make the following changes at home: _____
_____
_____
_____
_____.

I'll make the following changes at work: _____
_____
_____
_____
_____.

Once I make changes at home and
at work to remove whatever temptations
I can, dieting will be easier.

today's to-do list

Check off the tasks you've completed. For any item you haven't completed, record when you're going to complete it.

_____ I read my Advantages Response Card at least twice.

_____ I read other Response Cards as needed.

_____ I ate slowly, sitting down and noticing every bite.

Circle one: Every time   Most of the time   Some of the time

_____ I gave myself credit when I engaged in helpful dieting behaviors.

Circle one: Every time   Most of the time   Some of the time

_____ I made changes at home.

_____ I made changes at work.

chapter 6

Week 2

Get Set: Prepare to Diet

Welcome to Week 2. By the end of this week, you'll be better equipped to start a diet than you've ever been before. Are you starting to get the idea that this time is going to be different? Are you starting to understand why, this time, you're going to be able to lose excess weight and keep it off for your lifetime?

Before I tell you what you're going to learn this week, though, take a minute to think about how you've already changed as a result of the tasks in Week 1. *What do you know now that you didn't know before?* For example, did you know a week ago that it's crucially important for you to review at least a couple of times a day all of the reasons that you have for losing weight, to choose a healthy diet (and have a backup plan), to sit down and eat slowly and mindfully *every time,* to give yourself credit *continually* for using helpful eating behaviors, and to catch and respond to sabotaging thoughts that interfere with doing these essential tasks? Do you now understand the importance of using Cognitive Therapy techniques to help you follow your diet and use good eating habits? It's the difference in your thinking that's going to allow you to make permanent changes in your eating habits.

It's crucially important for you to *review* at
least a couple of times a day *all the reasons you
have for wanting to lose weight.*

How did Week 1 go for you? If you accomplished each day's task, then the likelihood that you're going to succeed on the Beck Diet Solution program is excellent.

Okay, on to Week 2. There's much more that goes into successful dieting than you may have realized. By the end of this week, you're going to know a great deal more. You're going to have more time and energy available for dieting, to be able to motivate yourself to exercise, to understand the importance of setting a short-term weight-loss goal, and to differentiate between and tolerate hunger and cravings. It'll be so wonderful once you find out—once and for all—that you never have to be concerned about feeling hungry or compelled to eat.

The Cognitive Therapy techniques you'll discover during Week 2 are designed to make the initial weeks of dieting go as smoothly as possible. As soon as you learn these additional skills, you'll have confidence that this time you'll succeed.

day 8
Create Time and Energy

Dieting takes a commitment that goes beyond eating differently. For starters, you'll need time to plan meals, to make lists, to shop for food, and to cook. You'll need to eat slowly, to exercise, and to read your Response Cards. It all takes fortitude and mental energy, especially if and when sabotaging thoughts get in the way.

Don't assume that this time and energy will magically make itself available to you. If you're like most people, your days may already be very busy with work, family responsibilities, housework, social events, volunteer work, and other commitments. Most dieters I've counseled over the years couldn't consistently find the time they needed to follow their diets until they *created* the time. In other words, they needed to look at their calendars and—in writing—schedule in time for dieting. Often, this meant decreasing, delegating, or eliminating some tasks and activities.

Today, I'd like you to do the same. Not only will there be a tangible benefit, but also there'll be a symbolic benefit: You'll be saying, in effect, *Yes, I get it ... This is going to take work, but I'm willing to do what it takes to lose weight ... It will be worth it.*

The first step in this process is figuring out how much time you'll need for dieting—at least initially, until you're in the swing of things. If possible, sit down with your diet coach and take a look at the suggested meals and recipes on the diet you've chosen. Think about the food you'll need for meals and snacks. This is important. If the food you planned to eat isn't readily available when you need it, you might opt for something else instead. Figure out how much time it will take in your day and week to:

- Plan your meals.
- Shop for the food you'll need.
- Prepare your meals.
- Sit down and eat your meals slowly.
- Exercise.
- Complete and check off the tasks on your daily to-do lists.

When Ben, a single guy in his mid-20s, reviewed his daily routine, he recognized that he'd have to make some changes to fit all these things into his schedule. He usually skipped breakfast and frequently snacked instead of eating a healthful lunch. Then he'd grab fast food for dinner. He thought about what he'd have to do to follow his diet and wrote the schedule on the facing page in his diet notebook.

How did Ben find the time? He did some problem solving. For one thing, he got out of bed a little earlier each weekday. He didn't particularly like doing this at first, but his desire to lose weight trumped his desire for that extra time in bed. Instead of always sitting on the couch watching TV, he watched some programs while he was preparing his meals. He cut down the time he spent on the computer by a few minutes each evening so he could plan meals for the next day and do other program tasks. Since he was particularly rushed on Tuesdays and Thursdays—he played basketball after work—Ben decided to bring his game clothes to work and change there instead of going home. He also decided to bring a substantial snack so he wouldn't be starving when the game was over. Ben quickly got used to his new routine and, before long, didn't have to keep a written schedule. His dieting activities became automatic.

For Lauri, Friday dinners were usually such a struggle because she was worn out from the work week. Although Lauri would have preferred to cook for her family on Fridays, she reluctantly recognized that it made more sense for her to buy prepared food to serve them. She was then able to reserve her energy for the many activities she had to do on weekends: attend her kids' sporting events, catch up with household tasks, and keep up with her busy social schedule. Lauri also negotiated with her husband to do more child care so she'd have time to properly prepare meals for her family and herself.

WEEKDAYS:
7:15–8:00 a.m. Prepare breakfast and lunch; eat breakfast.
5:30–6:00 p.m. Drive to the market [or to a favorite take-
    out place] to pick up dinner OR heat up already prepared
    food.
8:00–8:30 p.m. Walk for half an hour.
8:45–9:00 p.m. Write out eating plan for tomorrow; do
    other program tasks.

SATURDAYS:
9:00–9:30 a.m. Prepare and eat breakfast.
1:30–2:00 p.m. Prepare and eat lunch.
5:45–6:00 p.m. Write out eating plan for tomorrow; do
    other program tasks.

SUNDAYS:
8:00–8:30 a.m. Prepare and eat breakfast.
12:00–12:30 p.m. Prepare and eat lunch.
2:00–3:00 p.m. Shop for groceries.
4:00–6:00 p.m. Prepare Sunday dinner and freeze leftovers
    [for several meals]; chop salad vegetables [to eat during
    the week].
7:00–7:30 p.m. Walk for half an hour.
8:45–9:00 p.m. Write out eating plan for tomorrow; do
    other program tasks.

How to Find More Time

Now, I'd like you to get your calendar, appointment book, or PDA. If you don't have any of these, use My Scheduling Chart (page 101). When you fill it out, it should look like the one on page 100 that was created by Marie, a single mom. Fill in one chart for a typical weekday and another for a typical weekend or nonwork day.

   If you follow a fairly simple routine, you might be able to schedule in each program task, as Ben did. If your schedule is already pretty full, like Marie's, you might need some help in problem solving. You'll need to figure out how you can delegate, cut back, or eliminate certain activities. The first step is to see very clearly how you're currently spending your time.

Marie's Scheduling Chart

(a typical weekday)

Time	Activity
6:00 a.m.	Get up; eat breakfast.
6:30	Exercise.
7:00	Shower; get dressed.
7:30	Get kids up.
8:00	Give kids breakfast; clean up kitchen.
8:30	Drive to work.
9:00	Work.
9:30	
10:00	
10:30	
11:00	
11:30	
Noon	Eat lunch.
12:30 p.m.	Do errands.
1:00	Work.
1:30	
2:00	
2:30	
3:00	
3:30	
4:00	
4:30	
5:00	Drive home.
5:30	Help kids with homework.
6:00	Prepare dinner.
6:30	Eat dinner.
7:00	Do dishes; start a load of laundry.
7:30	Take kids to music lessons, do errands, shopping, etc.
8:00	
8:30	Get kids in bed.
9:00	Plan tomorrow's dinner; make lunches for everyone.
9:30	Pay bills, straighten up downstairs, finish laundry, etc.
10:00	E-mail or call friends.
10:30	Watch TV or read.
11:00	Go to bed.

My Scheduling Chart

Use this chart to fill in your daily schedule. If you work the night shift or follow a routine that is different from the one noted here, write in times that are appropriate to your situation.

Time	Activity
6:00 a.m.	
6:30	
7:00	
7:30	
8:00	
8:30	
9:00	
9:30	
10:00	
10:30	
11:00	
11:30	
Noon	
12:30 p.m.	
1:00	
1:30	
2:00	
2:30	
3:00	
3:30	
4:00	
4:30	
5:00	
5:30	
6:00	
6:30	
7:00	
7:30	
8:00	
8:30	
9:00	
9:30	
10:00	
10:30	
11:00	

Reducing Your Activities

Review your home and family responsibilities and decide which tasks you can delegate. For example, Sharon decided that she could get her teenagers to do after-dinner kitchen duty. They grumbled and moped at first and didn't do as good a job as Sharon would have, but the kitchen got cleaned nevertheless.

Delegating this activity allowed Sharon to leave the kitchen after dinner (eliminating the opportunity to nibble on food as she put it away) and gave her a chance to plan meals for the next day. She also was able to put her feet up for a few minutes and read the newspaper without interruption, which improved her mood and increased her mental energy—both important ingredients for being able to maintain motivation for dieting. She enjoyed this time to herself so much that she regretted not having delegated this task years earlier.

Next, you need to figure out which tasks you can cut back or eliminate. Jeremy really wanted to work on some home projects (painting his bedroom, cleaning the garage, gardening) on weekends, but he found he just didn't have the time or energy for the first couple of weeks of his diet to do all of these extra things and still be able to fit in exercise and healthy meal preparation. Because he knew losing weight was worth it, he decided to put off the first two projects and do only minimal yard work.

If you have trouble figuring out how to reduce your activities, making a priority chart can help. First, fill in your calendar or schedule chart with all your commitments for the coming week. Then divide these activities and tasks into three categories: essential, highly desirable, and desirable. Discuss with your diet coach just how important each task or activity really is. You'll probably find that many tasks you had previously thought of as essential are, in fact, just desirable and that you can put them on the back burner for a few weeks until dieting gets easier.

Here is how one dieter, Lisa, found a way to make time for weight loss in her life:

Lisa's Daily Activities

- Work: 8+ hours a day
- Being a mom (play with Hillary, read books to her, follow bedtime routine): 3 to 4 hours a day
- Household management (cooking, cleaning, bill paying): 1 to 2 hours a day
- Exercise or walk: 20 minutes a day
- Watch TV: 1 hour a day
- E-mail and surf the Internet: 1 hour a day
- Talk on the phone: half hour a day
- Volunteer with nonprofit group: 2 hours, twice a week

Lisa's Priority Chart

Essential Activities	Highly Desirable	Desirable
Some mom activities: get Hillary dressed, bathed, and fed; read for 15 min.; play/talk to her for 30 min.; bedtime routine	Watch some TV. Some mom activities: take Hillary for a walk, go to playground, read/play/talk to her more	Some mom activities: additional time for playing, reading, etc. Additional housework
Work		
	Other personal activities: bath instead of shower; long phone conversation with mom, sister, or best friend	Additional TV
Some housework: cook, do laundry, make beds, do dishes		Additional reading
		Additional e-mailing
Exercise or walk.		
	Additional housework	Surfing the Internet
Some personal activities: read for 20 min.; talk on the phone for 15 min.; e-mail for 15 min.	Shop for clothes.	Volunteer work
Do errands: shop for food.		
Prepare meals.		
Pay household bills.		

Once Lisa divided her activities into these broad categories, she could more easily see the advantage of temporarily cutting back on her volunteer work and TV viewing to make time for weight loss. When she explained to her husband why she needed to make extra time in her schedule, he was more willing (with some initial grumbling that she had to ignore) to take over some specific household chores. Lisa also decided to forgo a weekly manicure to free up some time and money to pay a cleaning service to tend to the house every other week.

Now, fill out My Priority Chart (page 104).

My Priority Chart

Essential Activities	Highly Desirable	Desirable

what are you thinking?

If you have difficulty devising or implementing the necessary changes in your schedule, you might have some preconceived ideas that are getting in your way.

Ann, for example, has a rule: *I shouldn't do anything that inconveniences others.* Therefore, she didn't even think of asking her husband to take over the grocery shopping, her mother to watch the kids so Ann could go to her support group, or her best friend to work with her on a community project.

Corrine has an unspoken rule: *I have to be the best mother possible.* Therefore, she didn't reduce such nonessential activities as picking up her youngsters at school (when they could have taken the school bus), taking them to every after-school activity they requested, and spending most of her free time doing things with them.

John also has a rule: *I have to keep my home in perfect order.* Since his wife was busy with other things (and just didn't care as much as he did about how their house looked), most of the household chores fell to him. It wasn't until John relaxed his standards that he finally created enough time and energy to devote to dieting.

If you, too, have set unreasonable rules for yourself, you might find it difficult to make changes. Ask yourself, *Do I truly have control over my schedule? Am I overburdened with responsibilities? Do I feel as if my life is just too complicated?* Don't decide that changes are impossible, though, until you've consulted with your diet coach. While your best shot at weight loss is to do the Beck Diet Solution program as suggested, you and your coach might decide that it's better for you to incorporate the steps more gradually.

Here are some other common sabotaging thoughts and helpful responses. If any are similar to your own thoughts, make Response Cards to help you.

Sabotaging Thought: I'm a spontaneous person. I don't like to schedule my time.
Helpful Response: To lose weight, I have to give up some spontaneity. I wish I didn't have to, but that's the way it is—at least for now. Until I've developed a routine, I can't rely on spontaneous shopping and spontaneous food preparation. But that doesn't mean that I can't be spontaneous in other ways.

Sabotaging Thought: I don't have the time to do the steps in this program.
Helpful Response: It might be more accurate to say that I'm not willing to *make* the time. If I had to get a blood transfusion every day to keep myself alive, obviously I'd *find* the time. While being overweight isn't necessarily life threatening, I still need to make a serious commitment if I want to diet successfully. I need to look at my Advantages Response Card again and judge whether I really want to lose weight.

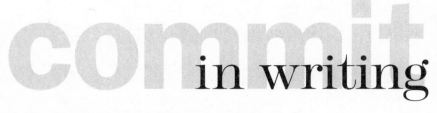

commit in writing

To make time and energy for dieting, I'm going to: _____
_____
_____
_____
_____.

> Once I accept the fact that dieting takes
> time and energy and I change my schedule
> accordingly, dieting will be easier.

today's to-do list

Have you completed all the tasks from Week 1?

- Do you already have your primary diet and backup diet?
- Have you thoroughly prepared your home and work environments?
- Have you had an initial conversation with your diet coach?

If not, add those tasks to your to-do list today, in addition to checking off the following items. For any item you haven't completed, record when you're going to complete it.

_____ I read my Advantages Response Card at least twice.

_____ I read my other Response Cards as needed.

_____ I ate slowly, sitting down and noticing every bite.

Circle one: Every time   Most of the time   Some of the time

_____ I gave myself credit when I engaged in helpful eating behaviors.

Circle one: Every time   Most of the time   Some of the time

_____ I looked at the week ahead, scheduled dieting into my calendar, and figured out how to eliminate or to cut back on some activities.

_____ I delegated some tasks (if needed) to other family members or asked a friend for help.

day 9
Select an Exercise Plan

Although many people attempt to lose weight through dieting alone, research clearly supports that your long-term success depends on also getting regular exercise. Results from the National Weight Control Registry—a study of thousands of participants who have lost more than 30 pounds and maintained that weight loss for at least a year—show that nearly 90 percent of dieters who lose weight and keep it off do so with a combination of diet and exercise; only 10 percent use diet alone, and 1 percent rely on only exercise.

Exercise has many diet- and non-diet-related benefits:

Exercise helps you stick with your diet. When you exercise, you say to yourself, *I'm serious about losing weight and getting in shape ... I'm willing to make a commitment, even if I start off very small ... I'm determined to succeed, once and for all.* Viewing exercise in this way can help you better commit to changing your eating, too, as this determination can carry over into your dieting efforts.

Exercise might help control appetite. Although study results are mixed, some physiologists believe that regular exercise helps to regulate the appetite-control system.

Exercise boosts mood and soothes stress. If you tend to eat in response to anxiety, frustration, and other negative emotions, exercise might provide a productive outlet.

Exercise burns calories. During exercise, your muscles burn calories at a faster rate than usual to power your movement. You also continue to burn calories at a slightly faster rate *after* a workout as your body recovers and rebuilds your muscles.

Exercise preserves muscle tissue. Usually, as you lose weight, you lose a combination of fat and muscle tissue. But exercise helps to preserve muscle tissue, so most of your weight loss comes from fat tissue.

Exercise builds confidence. As you increase your fitness, you're likely to feel better about yourself and your abilities. Researchers at the University of Houston in Texas found that students who participated in a six-week weight-training program reported feeling more positive about their appearance, less anxious about their bodies, and more confident in their abilities than students who didn't exercise.

Exercise makes you feel better physically. The more you move, the more you feel like moving. Regular exercise strengthens your lungs, heart, and other muscles, with the result that your daily activities (such as carrying bags of groceries or doing housework) feel less taxing. Because exercise can improve sleep, you might find that you have more energy as well.

Exercise improves your health and helps prevent disease. Studies have found a correlation between regular exercise and a reduced risk for heart disease, diabetes, and certain types of cancer.

How to Start

If you're not already doing so, you should engage in two kinds of exercise: spontaneous exercise (taking advantage of situations you're in to get more exercise) and planned exercise (setting a specific time to do a specific type of exercise).

Before starting an exercise program, check with your health-care provider. He or she will take your current state of health and weight into consideration and can then make suggestions or confirm that your choices are appropriate for you.

did you know?

The Centers for Disease Control report that only 17.5 percent of dieters combine dieting with exercise. No wonder it's so difficult for most people to lose weight, much less keep it off.

Spontaneous Exercise

You can start incorporating spontaneous exercise into your day right now. From today on, do the following:

- Always try to arrive at your destination ahead of time, so you can get off the bus or park far away and walk the extra distance.
- When you take an elevator, get off on the floor below your destination and walk up a flight of stairs. Over time, you might get off two floors early, then three, and so on.
- If you live in a two-story house, don't let things that need to be taken to another floor pile up; take each up right away.
- When you go to the mall, walk a full circuit before you start shopping. Whenever you find yourself waiting (such as at the doctor's office, at the airport, or at the hair salon), walk the concourses, the hallways, or the sidewalks outside.

To motivate yourself to do more spontaneous exercise, consider attaching to your belt a pedometer, a device that tracks the distance you cover on foot. You can buy a good pedometer for about $20 at sporting-goods stores, many fitness centers, or over the Internet. Wear the pedometer every day and note in your diet notebook how many steps you've taken. Challenge yourself to continually add more steps to your day and to track your progress.

Planned Exercise

Since exercising is not optional if you want to lose weight, be sure to choose a form of exercise that you like and can stick with. If you're not sure what you want to do, consult a friend or health-care professional (the latter is especially important if you have a health condition or have been sedentary for a long time). Try some of the exercises my patients ended up enjoying:

- Take a daily walk or run.
- Join a gym.
- Swim laps or do water aerobics.
- Exercise to a video tape, DVD, or TV fitness show.
- Play a sport.
- Hire a personal trainer.
- Participate in exercise or dance classes.

No matter what form of planned exercise you choose, start out at a reasonable level. It's not realistic to go from doing nothing to exercising 30 minutes a day. You'll just get sore muscles or possibly injure yourself—then you're likely to give up exercising completely.

If you've been relatively sedentary, start with walking five minutes every day until it feels relatively easy. Then gradually add a minute at a time to your walk. Remind yourself that even five minutes is better than zero minutes!

Solve Common Exercise Problems

Many health or lifestyle issues can make starting an exercise program more difficult, but they shouldn't rule out exercise. However, you might need to be creative. If you can't figure out a way to fit in exercise, consult your diet coach or consider what you'd tell a friend who came to you with the same problem. Though dieters have told me about many problems they initially thought were unsolvable, we were able to figure out solutions. Here are a few:

<u>Problem:</u> I have two small children who need constant supervision.
<u>Solutions:</u> Exercise at a fitness center that offers child care. Swap babysitting with another parent. Exercise with your children to a family fitness video, ride bikes, or walk. Exercise to a fitness DVD while your children play nearby.

<u>Problem:</u> I have physical limitations.
<u>Solutions:</u> Many people can swim or take a water fitness class. Others need to start with physical therapy. Consult your health-care provider for a referral to an appropriate program.

Problem: I don't have enough time.

Solutions: Schedule exercise into your appointment calendar. Consider which daily activities you can decrease or eliminate to make time for exercise. Consider getting up earlier and starting your day with exercise. Make exercise an essential activity, not an optional one.

Problem: I'm embarrassed to exercise where others will see me.

Solutions: Exercise at home to a fitness video or with a close friend who can provide moral support. Best of all, develop a more helpful mindset. Besides, who cares what others think? I've found that most exercisers are only concerned with their own activities. If they notice you at all, it'll be for only a brief moment; then they'll return their attention to what *they* are doing.

tip!

If you struggle to motivate yourself to exercise, ask a friend or official exercise coach (such as a personal trainer) to meet you for your exercise sessions. It's easy to let yourself down by skipping exercise, but it's much harder to let down a friend or trainer. Your coach can also work with you to help you overcome your physical and attitudinal difficulties.

Finalize Your Exercise Plans

If you currently exercise fewer than three times a week, your goal for today is to establish a more frequent exercise routine. Make arrangements to begin a planned exercise program as soon as possible. Meanwhile, set a time to take a walk every day—even if you can go for only five minutes—and put it in your daily appointment calendar or schedule.

Also think of all of the different ways you can work spontaneous exercise into each day. Write down your plan so you'll feel accountable.

what are you thinking?

Sabotaging thoughts will interfere with your ability to start and maintain an exercise program. Most are self-deluding or irrelevant, such as, *A lot of people don't exercise, so it's okay if I don't either.* If you find yourself resisting the idea of starting an exercise program, reread the benefits of exercise mentioned on pages 107–108. Which are important to you? Write them on a Response Card.

Use the following helpful responses to common sabotaging thoughts to create inspiration for making additional cards.

Sabotaging Thought: I don't want to exercise.
Helpful Response: I shouldn't go by whether I want to exercise. If I want to lose weight and keep it off, I *need* to exercise. There are also lots of other benefits to exercising. I might be making this into a much bigger deal than it really is. I can do this.

Sabotaging Thought: What's the use of walking for only five minutes?
Helpful Response: Walking for five minutes is better than walking for zero minutes. Exercise is essential, even if I don't do very much at first. I can build up the amount that I do over time, but I have to start somewhere.

Sabotaging Thought: I'm too busy to exercise.
Helpful Response: I have to make exercise a priority. If I needed to exercise each day to stay alive, I'd find the time. I might have to get up earlier in the morning to fit it in, but I shouldn't fool myself into thinking that exercise is optional.

Sabotaging Thought: It isn't worth it to me to exercise.
Helpful Response: Research shows that exercise is essential for most people to lose weight and to maintain their weight loss. If I want the benefits of being thinner, I have to exercise.

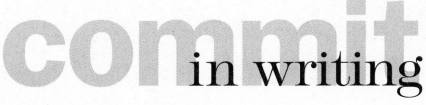

commit in writing

The spontaneous exercise I'm going to do daily is: _____
_____
_____
_____ .

The planned exercise I'm going to do several times a week is: _____
_____
_____
_____ .

> Once I accept that exercise is
> essential and start doing it consistently,
> dieting will be easier.

today's to-do list

Check off the tasks you've completed. For any item you haven't completed, record when you're going to complete it.

_____ I read my Advantages Response Card at least twice.

_____ I read my other Response Cards as needed.

_____ I ate slowly, sitting down and noticing every bite.

Circle one: Every time   Most of the time   Some of the time

_____ I gave myself credit when I engaged in helpful eating behaviors.

Circle one: Every time   Most of the time   Some of the time

_____ I did at least one spontaneous exercise today.

_____ I investigated the possibilities of a planned exercise program.

_____ I scheduled exercise time in my appointment book.

_____ I did planned exercise.

day 10
Set a Realistic Goal

Setting a goal for yourself can be a great motivator—but you can easily become overwhelmed if you set a goal that seems too daunting or will take too long to achieve. Don't fall into that trap.
What is your goal?

- To get to a certain weight
- To fit into a particular size of clothing
- To look the way you looked when you were younger

It's natural to want to set a long-term goal. In reality, though, we don't yet know whether your goal is reasonable for you. I also don't want you to become anxious thinking how far you have to go. Instead, I'd like you to set a short-term goal to lose 5 pounds.

You probably want to lose more than that, of course. So once you lose 5 pounds, set a new goal to lose 5 more pounds, and so on. Each time you lose 5 pounds, celebrate. Call a friend or your diet coach, and celebrate together. Or buy yourself something you can afford that you've wanted for a while.

One woman I counseled bought an inexpensive charm for her charm bracelet every time she reached a new 5-pound goal. Consider indulging yourself in some non-food-related way—with a tennis lesson or a massage, for example. It's important to celebrate your small successes along the way, rather than waiting until you've lost a lot of weight to feel good about your efforts.

Now, let's talk about the *rate* at which you should try to lose weight. Although you probably don't want to hear this, the answer is the slower the better. During the first week, you might lose several pounds. This isn't unusual since at the start of a diet most weight loss actually comes from water and not from fat. You probably won't continue losing at that rate, though, so don't get discouraged later on.

> Although you probably don't want to hear this, *the rate at which you should try to lose weight is the slower the better.*

In fact, there is no long-term benefit to losing weight too quickly. And there is a major disadvantage: When you suddenly decrease the amount of food that you eat, your body responds in a protective manner by slowing your metabolism. It's your body's natural response to protect you from starvation.

Weight-loss specialists agree that your goal should be to lose no more than 1 to 2 pounds a week. But it's fine if you lose only a half pound a week on average.

what are you thinking?

Do you still have a goal to reach a specific number on the scale one day? Are you hoping to lose weight very quickly?

Read the following sabotaging thoughts and responses to help you commit to 5-pound incremental goals.

Sabotaging Thought: I won't be satisfied unless I get down to my "ideal" weight. I don't deserve credit until I get down to that weight.
Helpful Response: I have to learn to be happy with smaller steps along the way. Celebrating 5-pound losses will boost my mood and confidence.

Sabotaging Thought: Losing only 1 to 2 pounds a week is much too slow!
Helpful Response: How much will it matter a few years from now how long it took? I need to remind myself why it's important to lose weight slowly. My long-term success depends on it.

commit in writing

My first weight-loss goal will be: _____
_____.

(I hope you wrote, "to lose 5 pounds.")

> Once I accept the fact that I should
> focus on losing 5 pounds at a time,
> dieting will be easier.

today's to-do list

Check off the tasks you've completed. For any item you haven't completed, record when you're going to complete it.

_____ I read my Advantages Response Card at least twice.

_____ I read my other Response Cards as needed.

_____ I ate slowly, sitting down and noticing every bite.

Circle one: Every time   Most of the time   Some of the time

_____ I gave myself credit when I engaged in helpful eating behaviors.

Circle one: Every time   Most of the time   Some of the time

_____ I did spontaneous exercise.

Circle one: Every opportunity   Some of the time   Once or twice   Not at all

_____ I did planned exercise.

_____ I set a goal to lose 5 pounds.

day 11
Differentiate Between Hunger, Desire, and Cravings

Almost every dieter I've worked with has had difficulty distinguishing between true hunger (when you've fasted for several hours and your stomach is empty), a desire to eat (not being particularly hungry but eating because there is food around), and a craving (a physiological and emotionally intense urge to eat). Interestingly, many of them initially thought they *could* tell the difference. What about you?

Think about times in the past when you've leisurely finished a rather large meal, perhaps when eating out at a restaurant or during a family celebration. I wonder if you ever had such thoughts as, *I'm still hungry ... I think I'll have seconds ... I'm hungry for dessert.*

If so, you confused hunger with a desire to eat. Today's task will help you figure out when you're truly hungry, so you can tell yourself, *Okay, I've finished the food I planned to eat for this meal, and I'm still hungry ... But that's okay ... It might take my brain 20 minutes to send a message to my body that I'm full ... I'll wait to see how I feel in 20 minutes.*

Or you might try saying to yourself, *Okay, I'm hungry, no big deal, I'm going to eat again in ___ hours ... Here's a chance to strengthen my resistance muscle* (described, along with the giving-in muscle, on page 29).

Or think to yourself, *I'm not hungry ... I just want to eat more ... But I'm not going to because I don't want to strengthen my giving-in muscle.*

Monitor Your Hunger

How do you know when you're really hungry? Think about three recent occasions when the following occurred:

- You hadn't eaten for many hours and really felt ravenous. That empty sensation in your stomach, often accompanied by stomach rumblings, was *hunger.*
- You ate a big meal and yet you still wanted to continue to eat more. That was a *desire.*
- You had a very strong urge to eat, which was accompanied by a feeling of tension and an unpleasant yearning sensation in your mouth, throat, or body. That was a *craving.*

To better differentiate between these sensations, pick a day to note what you experience before, during, and after you eat.

Most dieters have difficulty
distinguishing between *true hunger,*
a desire to eat, and a craving.

Before you sit down to eat each meal and snack, notice how your stomach feels. Write a description of this feeling in My Hunger Monitoring Chart on page 118. Also, rate your stomach hunger on a scale of 0 to 10, with 0 being not hungry at all and 10 being the hungriest that you've ever felt.

Halfway through the meal, notice how your stomach feels. Write a description of this sensation in the chart. Then rate your hunger, using the same 0 to 10 scale.

Rate your hunger again once you've finished eating. Notice your thoughts: Do you still want to eat more? Do you feel a physical sensation in your stomach? Is it more in your mouth or throat? What does it feel like? How strong are your sensations? Do you want to eat a specific food (which probably means you're desiring or craving) or will any food do (which probably means you're still hungry)? Describe the sensations in the chart.

Twenty minutes after you've finished eating, rate your hunger and then describe any physical sensations or desire to eat that you're experiencing in the chart.

The sample chart below was filled out by Pamela, one of the dieters I counseled:

Pamela's Hunger Monitoring Chart

Time	How My Stomach Feels	Strength of Hunger (0–10)
Before dinner	Very empty, a little bit of growling	8
Midway through dinner	A little fuller	5
Immediately after dinner	Mildly full, but want to eat seconds; feel an urge in my mouth and throat	2
20 minutes after dinner	Full, satisfied, glad I didn't eat too much	0

My Hunger Monitoring Chart

Use this chart to complete today's task, with 0 being not hungry and 10 being the hungriest you've ever felt.

Time	How My Stomach Feels	Strength of Hunger (0–10)
Before breakfast		
Midway through breakfast		
Immediately after breakfast		
20 minutes after breakfast		
Before lunch		
Midway through lunch		
Immediately after lunch		
20 minutes after lunch		
Before dinner		
Midway through dinner		
Immediately after dinner		
20 minutes after dinner		

After a day of paying attention to the sensations in your abdomen and body, you'll be better able to distinguish between "hungry" and "not hungry." If you're still not sure, repeat the task—as many times as necessary—and discuss your findings with your diet coach. Whenever you know your stomach is full but you still want to eat, start labeling this state as desire or a craving.

tip!
If it has been anywhere from 20 minutes to up to 3 hours since you've eaten a reasonable-sized meal, remind yourself that any urge to eat is probably due to a desire to eat, not to hunger.

what are you thinking?

Below are some common sabotaging thoughts and responses. Make Response Cards for any that ring true for you.

Sabotaging Thought: I don't need to do this. I know the difference between hunger and craving.

Helpful Response: I might know the difference on an intellectual level, but it's still important for me to experience the difference on a physical level. Chances are, I probably sometimes label a craving as hunger. It's very important for me to do this exercise so I'll know whether I really am too hungry too often (which is a problem I'll need to solve) or whether I really am craving (which is a sensation I'll learn to tolerate).

Sabotaging Thought: This task is too much trouble. I don't feel like doing it.

Helpful Response: It doesn't take very much time or energy. Why not try it and see what happens?

Sabotaging Thought: Why do I need to know the difference? I'm just going to follow my diet plan anyway.

Helpful Response: When I get to maintenance, I can be more flexible with my eating if I eat only in response to hunger. Unless I practice differentiating between hunger and craving now, I won't be able to do this successfully and I'll gain weight.

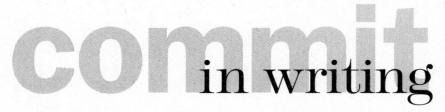

commit in writing

To learn to figure out when I'm really hungry, I'm going to: _____
_____
_____
_____ .

Once I learn to tell the difference between hunger and craving, dieting will be easier.

today's to-do list

Check off the tasks you've completed. For any item you haven't completed, record when you're going to complete it.

_____ I read my Advantages Response Card at least twice today.

_____ I read my other Response Cards as needed.

_____ I ate slowly, sitting down and noticing every bite.

Circle one: Every time   Most of the time   Some of the time

_____ I gave myself credit when I engaged in helpful eating behaviors.

Circle one: Every time   Most of the time   Some of the time

_____ I did spontaneous exercise.

Circle one: Every opportunity   Some of the time   Once or twice   Not at all

_____ I did planned exercise.

_____ I rated (or decided on a future day to rate) my hunger on My Hunger Monitoring Chart.

day 12
Practice Hunger Tolerance

Yesterday, you learned the differences between hunger, desire, and cravings. Today's task is a little tougher. You're going to learn how to tolerate hunger.

Are you concerned about being hungry? When I ask dieters this question, they invariably answer no—initially. But when I suggest today's exercise, most of them become uncomfortable. Some have said, "I'm not *concerned* about it. I just don't *want* to be hungry." It turned out, though, that there was more to it: They were anxious. *At some level, they didn't know if they could actually tolerate being hungry.*

When people who struggle with dieting get hungry, they often feel hunger pangs intensely. The sensations can feel like an emergency. All their attention gets focused on how uncomfortable they feel—and when and where they can get food. They begin to think they won't be able to stand feeling that way.

If you've had similar experiences, it's important to learn that you *can* tolerate hunger. Once you effectively convince yourself of this, hunger won't seem like such a big deal. When you're hungry but it's not time for a meal or a snack, you'll be able to say to yourself, *Oh, well, I wish I could eat now, but it's okay ... I can wait.*

You'll then be able to turn your attention to other things, and the hunger pangs will gradually diminish. If you've never allowed yourself to feel hungry or very hungry, you might not believe me when I tell you that if you're hungry and don't respond immediately by eating, then your hunger will definitely subside.

Today's task will help you see that you *can* tolerate hunger and that it comes and goes. Today or one day very soon (you can choose what works best with your schedule), I'd like you to purposely skip lunch. (Don't do this if a medical condition, such as diabetes, requires you to eat regularly.) Doing so will help you realize that *hunger is not an emergency.* In fact, I think you'll find it's not nearly as uncomfortable a sensation as you now believe.

If you fear hunger, you might routinely eat to avoid the feeling. You might never have learned that it's okay to feel hungry, or you might never have developed skills to help you withstand hunger. Purposely skipping a meal will prove something to you: You definitely don't have to eat when you're hungry. Just because you want to eat doesn't mean you always should. This is one of the most important things you need to learn to lose excess weight and to keep it off!

You definitely don't have to eat when you're hungry. Just because you want to eat doesn't mean you always should.

What to Do

Pick a day this week to practice hunger tolerance. If you think it'll be challenging, choose a day when you know you'll be busy and you predict you won't be faced with difficult eating triggers. Many of the dieters I've counseled initially tried this experiment on a workday. A structured routine helped them refrain from eating until dinnertime.

To help you put the discomfort of hunger in perspective, reflect on past non-hunger-related experiences that were uncomfortable. Use My Discomfort Scale on the facing page and fill in several points, with 0 representing a situation in which you experienced no discomfort and 10 representing a situation in which you had the most extreme discomfort you've ever experienced.

Below is a scale that Carolyn, a dieter I counseled, filled out:

Carolyn's Discomfort Scale

Discomfort Level	Situation
0	Sitting around watching a sitcom right after dinner
1	
2	
3	When I went on a job interview
4	
5	Waiting for a medical test
6	
7	
8	When I had root canal surgery
9	
10	When I broke my leg

My Discomfort Scale

Zero represents a situation in which you experienced no discomfort at all, and 10 represents a situation in which you had extreme discomfort.

Discomfort Level	Situation
0	
1	
2	
3	
4	
5	
6	
7	
8	
9	
10	

You'll use this scale to rate how uncomfortable your hunger gets on the day you decide to skip lunch. Make sure to create this scale; you're going to need it to complete tomorrow's task, too.

Going Hungry

On the day you practice feeling hungry, on every hour you're going to track how uncomfortable you feel on My Hunger Discomfort Chart. At right is an example of how Norma, a dieter I counseled, filled in her chart. Doing this exercise helped her realize that her hunger never got above a 4 in discomfort and that she absolutely was able to tolerate it.

On the day you choose, eat breakfast and then purposely *don't eat again* until dinner. At the time you normally eat lunch, figure out how uncomfortable (not how hungry) you are and write your rating on My Hunger Discomfort Chart. Then every hour or so between lunch and dinner, rate how strong your discomfort is at that very moment. Also reflect on how the previous hour went and record how high or low your discomfort was.

Norma's Hunger Discomfort Chart

Time	Current Level of Discomfort 0–10	Range of Discomfort in Last Hour 0–10
noon	3	0–3
1:00 p.m.	2	0–3
2:00	0	0–4
3:00	3	0–3
4:00	4	0–4
5:00	3	0–4
6:00	3	0–4

My Hunger Discomfort Chart

Time	Current Level of Discomfort 0–10	Range of Discomfort in Last Hour 0–10
noon		
1:00 p.m.		
2:00		
3:00		
4:00		
5:00		
6:00		

what are you thinking?

During your hunger experiment, you might need to repeatedly confront sabotaging thoughts, such as, *I don't want to keep doing this ... This is too uncomfortable.* Remind yourself that there have been times in your life when you've been hungry but survived: when you fasted for a medical procedure or religious holiday, when you couldn't eat because you were delayed in traffic, or when service was extremely slow in a restaurant. You'll always survive because *hunger is never an emergency.*

If these kinds of thoughts overpower you and lead you to eat before dinner, try this experiment again and again, each time increasing the amount of time that elapses before you eat. If your fear of hunger is too strong, you might need to conquer it more gradually.

Here are some common sabotaging thoughts experienced by dieters who struggle with tolerating hunger. Make Response Cards to read whenever you need them.

Sabotaging Thought: I should eat when I'm hungry. Isn't that what everyone does?
Helpful Response: Most people don't eat every time they're hungry. They wait until their next meal. I need to learn that skill, too.

Sabotaging Thought: Why should I deliberately make myself feel uncomfortable by skipping lunch?
Helpful Response: I need to experience hunger to decrease my fear of it. This experiment will help reduce my anxiety about hunger in the future. The best way to get over my fear is to face it. This experiment will strengthen me for the next time I'm hungry and it's not time to eat.

commit in writing

The day I'm going to do my hunger experiment is: _____.

Once I get over my intolerance of
hunger, dieting will be easier.

today's to-do list

Check off the tasks you've completed. For any item you haven't completed, record when you're going to complete it.

_____ I read my Advantages Response Card at least twice today.

_____ I read my other Response Cards as needed.

_____ I ate slowly, sitting down and noticing every bite.

Circle one: Every time   Most of the time   Some of the time

_____ I gave myself credit when I engaged in helpful eating behaviors.

Circle one: Every time   Most of the time   Some of the time

_____ I did spontaneous exercise.

Circle one: Every opportunity   Some of the time   Once or twice   Not at all

_____ I did planned exercise.

_____ I planned a day to skip lunch in order to learn that I can tolerate feeling hungry.

day 13
Overcome Cravings

I once saw a cartoon depicting a woman looking panicky in her kitchen while food from cabinets, the countertop, table, and refrigerator were talking to her, with balloon text saying, "Eat me! Eat me! Eat me!" Have you ever had a similar experience, when it seemed that food was calling out to you? I certainly have and so has everyone I've counseled. The good news is that even though foods might continue to call out to you, you *can* stay in control.

Cravings usually peak within the first few weeks of your diet. Once you limit or stop eating the foods you crave (usually fast food, sweets, salty snacks, and the like), your cravings for those foods will diminish significantly. Today, you'll learn how to deal with cravings effectively and decisively.

If you've successfully dieted in the past, you might remember how wonderful it feels when you stop experiencing intense cravings. To weaken the intensity and reduce the frequency of cravings, however, you have to *stop giving in to them*. People who struggle with dieting usually find that they don't limit themselves to just a small taste of the food they crave; even though they try to eat just a little, they end up eating a lot. Have you also found that cravings don't usually go away by trying to satisfy them with just a taste?

Waiting out a craving increases your ability to tolerate cravings and also increases your confidence that you can do so. The more often you wait out your cravings, the less intense and less frequent they'll be in the future. Eventually, you'll experience a craving, and, instead of feeling bad, you'll feel good. You'll spontaneously say to yourself, *This is great ... I'm feeling a craving, but I know I can tolerate it and it'll go away ... It's great that I'm tolerating it!* Instead of feeling deprived, you'll feel good—proud, strong, confident, in control. Dieting will get so much easier.

To get to that point, however, you first must learn how to respond to your cravings. This is actually simpler than many people realize. Cravings start to diminish the moment you decide you're absolutely *not* going to stray from your diet. They increase when you're indecisive about whether or not to eat.

To weaken the intensity and reduce
the frequency of cravings, *you have to
stop giving in to them.*

Today, you'll learn how to prove to yourself that you don't have to give in to cravings and eat to make them disappear. You can take control and make them go away. First, you'll collect information about your cravings so you can demonstrate this to yourself. Then you'll learn anti-craving techniques.

Discovering that you can tolerate cravings is one of the most important things you need to learn to lose weight and keep it off!

How to Measure Your Cravings

Your next craving might surface today, tomorrow, or as long as a few weeks from now. When it does, I'd like you to fill out My Cravings Rating Chart on the facing page with the following information:

- How long your craving lasts
- How uncomfortable it is on the discomfort scale (0–10)
- Which anti-craving techniques you used

When Francine, a dieter I counseled, filled out her Cravings Rating Chart, she discovered that her cravings weren't as painful as she had predicted. She also found that the sooner she convinced herself that she wasn't going to eat and got involved in other activities, the sooner the craving went away. This is what her chart looked like:

Francine's Cravings Rating Chart

Day/Time	Monday, 3 p.m.	Monday, 7 p.m.	Monday, 9:30 p.m.
How uncomfortable did the craving get on my discomfort scale? (0–10)	6	3	2
How long did it last?	10 min.	4 min.	2 min.
What anti-craving techniques did I try?	Did the mindset techniques; left the room; did relaxed breathing; got back to work.	Did the mindset techniques; drank a glass of water; e-mailed friends.	Did the mindset techniques; put leftover food down garbage disposal.

My Cravings Rating Chart

Use My Discomfort Scale (page 123), which you filled out yesterday, to help you rate how uncomfortable your cravings really are.

Day/Time			
How uncomfortable did the craving get on my discomfort scale? (0–10)			
How long did it last?			
What anti-craving techniques did I try?			
Day/Time			
How uncomfortable did the craving get on my discomfort scale? (0–10)			
How long did it last?			
What anti-craving techniques did I try?			

As part of this exercise, you'll fill out My Cravings Rating Chart, but first you need to learn anti-craving strategies, including mindset techniques and behavioral techniques.

The emotionally painful part about a craving is the struggle you feel. Once you can say to yourself with total conviction, NO CHOICE, the craving will diminish.

Anti-Craving Strategies

Mindset Techniques

You can take a number of steps to respond to your next craving. The first five steps help you prepare your mindset, and you should use the following every time you have a craving:

1. Label it. Tell yourself, *This feeling is just a craving … It's uncomfortable and intense, but (like hunger) it's not an emergency.*

2. Stand firm. Tell yourself that you're absolutely *not* going to eat the food that you're craving. Remind yourself that you truly don't want to strengthen your giving-in muscle and weaken your resistance muscle. Ask yourself whether giving in to this craving will be worth the momentary pleasure you'll get from eating. Think about how giving in can undermine your confidence.

3. Don't give yourself a choice. The emotionally painful part about a craving is the struggle you feel. Once you can tell yourself with total conviction, *NO CHOICE,* and do something else, the craving will diminish. (You'll read more about this on Day 16 on pages 149–152.) It won't go away, though, if you waver or say to yourself, *This is so intense, I don't know if I can stand it.* Of course, you can stand it! It might be uncomfortable, but nothing bad will happen if you withstand it. In fact, in a few moments, you're going to be so proud of yourself!

4. Imagine the aftermath of giving in. Go ahead and think about eating the food you're craving. Imagine it in your mouth. How many seconds does it take to eat it? How many seconds do you feel pleasure? Now visualize *the rest of the picture*—the part of the experience you usually don't think about until it's too late. Picture yourself feeling weak and out of control. See yourself feeling upset, giving up, continuing to eat more and more, feeling worse and worse. Do you start to feel heavier in your body or more heavy-hearted? As you become upset in the image, remind yourself how many times you've given in before, how you promised yourself you wouldn't do it again, and how hopeless you felt.

Now that you've seen the entire picture, which seems better: eating or not eating?

5. Remind yourself why you want to learn to withstand cravings. Read your Advantages Response Card. You won't be able to attain the wonderful benefits of losing weight unless you tolerate your cravings. If you continue to give in to them, you'll always be at risk for gaining weight.

Behavioral Techniques

If you're still tempted to eat something you shouldn't after you've done all five mindset techniques, then try as many of the behavioral techniques below as you need:

1. Distance yourself from the food you crave. When you experience a craving because you see or smell food, you might be able to move that food to an inconvenient place (where you can't see it) or to get rid of it (give it away, throw it away, or put it down the disposal).

If you can't remove the food from your immediate presence, you might be able to remove *yourself* from the scene. Leave the room, go to another part of the room, go to the restroom (and read your Response Cards), or go outside.

2. Drink a no- or low-calorie beverage. Thirst can mask as hunger and trigger you to eat. Consider drinking club soda, water with lemon, diluted juice (if your plan allows it), or another low-calorie drink.

3. Relax. You can teach your body how to relax in a variety of ways. Your library or bookstore has tapes and books on relaxation techniques. One simple relaxation technique involves focusing on your breathing: Breathe in and out of your nose, slowly counting to four as you inhale and again to four as you exhale. Use very shallow breaths; don't let your chest rise and fall. Set a timer and keep up this technique for a full three minutes. At the end of the three minutes, you should feel calmer and more in control of your cravings.

4. Distract yourself. Do you remember a time when a natural distraction interrupted your craving and you later were glad you hadn't eaten? Maybe a friend called, the dog insisted on taking you for a walk, or your boss came to discuss something with you? By the time you finished what you had to do, your craving had weakened or passed. You focused your attention on something else.

> When you experience a craving
> because you see or smell food, move the food
> to an inconvenient place or get rid of it—or
> *remove yourself from the scene.*

My Distraction Activities Chart

Rate each distraction on a scale of 0 to 10, with 0 meaning this activity didn't help at all and 10 meaning this activity helped completely.

Distraction Activity	Effectiveness (0–10)										
	0	1	2	3	4	5	6	7	8	9	10
Brush your teeth.	○	○	○	○	○	○	○	○	○	○	○
Polish your nails.	○	○	○	○	○	○	○	○	○	○	○
Reread parts of this book.	○	○	○	○	○	○	○	○	○	○	○
Call a friend or your diet coach.	○	○	○	○	○	○	○	○	○	○	○
Talk to a neighbor or coworker.	○	○	○	○	○	○	○	○	○	○	○
Go to a store.	○	○	○	○	○	○	○	○	○	○	○
Play with a child or pet.	○	○	○	○	○	○	○	○	○	○	○
Ride your bicycle.	○	○	○	○	○	○	○	○	○	○	○
Go for a walk or exercise.	○	○	○	○	○	○	○	○	○	○	○
Read or write e-mail.	○	○	○	○	○	○	○	○	○	○	○
Take a bath or shower.	○	○	○	○	○	○	○	○	○	○	○
Do a crafts project.	○	○	○	○	○	○	○	○	○	○	○
Put together a puzzle.	○	○	○	○	○	○	○	○	○	○	○
Practice a musical instrument.	○	○	○	○	○	○	○	○	○	○	○
Tinker with the car.	○	○	○	○	○	○	○	○	○	○	○
Work in the garden or yard.	○	○	○	○	○	○	○	○	○	○	○
Put photographs in an album.	○	○	○	○	○	○	○	○	○	○	○
Do a specific chore (such as clean out a desk drawer).	○	○	○	○	○	○	○	○	○	○	○
Putter around the house (such as change lightbulbs, replace smoke detector batteries, etc.).	○	○	○	○	○	○	○	○	○	○	○
Surf the Internet (keep a running list of things you've always wanted to look up and save them for these times).	○	○	○	○	○	○	○	○	○	○	○
Write additional distraction techniques here:											
_____	○	○	○	○	○	○	○	○	○	○	○
_____	○	○	○	○	○	○	○	○	○	○	○
_____	○	○	○	○	○	○	○	○	○	○	○
_____	○	○	○	○	○	○	○	○	○	○	○
_____	○	○	○	○	○	○	○	○	○	○	○

You'll probably initially find that you need a pretty strong distraction to get your attention off the food you crave. Many dieters try to distract themselves by watching TV or reading. I've found that most of the time these kinds of activities are just not compelling enough. If they work for you, that's fine. But you'll also find a number of activities that are potentially more distracting in My Distraction Activities Chart on the facing page. Try as many as you can and assess how effectively each works. Rate each on a scale of 0 to 10.

After you've tried a number of techniques, make a list of the most helpful ones in your diet notebook, starting with the activities that were most effective. As you discover additional possibilities, try them out and add them to your list.

As you follow your diet plan and tolerate craving after craving, you'll find that cravings definitely diminish. You won't have to do battle whenever you see your favorite foods. It'll be such a relief to know that you can resist foods you haven't planned to eat, even if the urge to eat is strong.

what are you thinking?

The following are typical sabotaging thoughts with helpful responses. Make Response Cards for any you think apply to you.

Sabotaging Thought: The next time I have a craving, I won't be able to tolerate it.
Helpful Response: I couldn't tolerate cravings in the past, but now I have lots of anti-craving techniques that I can use, which will make the craving go away. Besides, the discomfort of cravings is mild compared to the discomfort I felt when _____.
I tolerated that, and I can certainly tolerate cravings.

Sabotaging Thought: I know myself. The next time I have a craving I won't want to control myself.
Helpful Response: That's probably true. But I can keep reminding myself that I don't want to be at the mercy of my cravings forever. To get rid of them, I'm always going to have to do one of two things: either give in and eat and never lose the weight I want or use the anti-craving techniques so often that I just won't have many cravings anymore. Once I find out these techniques really work, I'll be able to wait out my cravings so much more easily. I'll be glad when I get to the point where I don't have to be worried when I go to a party or eat out. I'll know for sure that I can tolerate these urges.

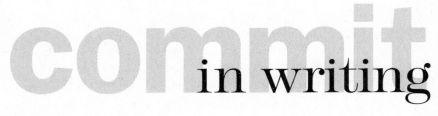

commit in writing

When I have a craving, I'll: _____
_____
_____
_____
_____.

Once I stop giving in to cravings and
they become much weaker and less frequent,
dieting will be easier.

today's to-do list

Check off the tasks you've completed. For any item you haven't completed, record when you're going to complete it.

_____ I read my Advantages Response Card at least twice today.

_____ I read my other Response Cards as needed.

_____ I ate slowly, sitting down and noticing every bite.

        Circle one: Every time   Most of the time   Some of the time

_____ I gave myself credit when I engaged in helpful eating behaviors.

        Circle one: Every time   Most of the time   Some of the time

_____ I did spontaneous exercise.

        Circle one: Every opportunity   Some of the time   Once or twice   Not at all

_____ I did planned exercise.

_____ I tolerated hunger.

_____ I planned how I'll tolerate cravings.

_____ I tolerated a craving.

day 14
Plan for Tomorrow

If you're not already dieting, you'll start tomorrow! If you already started dieting, you'll still need to do today's task.

Today, you're going to write a food plan that includes *everything* you're going to eat tomorrow. And, tomorrow, you'll check off whatever you eat that's on the plan and write down any food you eat that isn't on the plan.

You'll continue to plan and monitor your eating in writing every day for many weeks and months, possibly until you've lost all the weight you want—and maybe even beyond.

Okay, I can almost hear your sabotaging thoughts. Writing a plan and monitoring what you eat is the single task the people I've counseled have most often resisted. You might be thinking the same kinds of things they've said to me, such as:

- *I don't really have to do that, do I?*
- *It's so much trouble. I don't want to do it.*
- *That means I can't just eat whatever I feel like eating.*

Writing and monitoring are *very* important, and if you're like most of the people I've worked with, I think you'll find that the idea of doing them is much more burdensome than the reality.

Planning what you eat is essential. It helps you to do the following:

- Think about how you're going to get and prepare the food on your eating plan.
- Remember what you're supposed to eat and when. If you don't plan ahead, you put yourself in the tougher situation of solving problems in the moment. When you feel hungry and look in your refrigerator for something to eat, you might not come up with a diet-friendly solution.
- Eliminate spontaneous eating. Spontaneous eating—the little nibbles of snacks, leftovers, and other food—is often what keeps dieters from losing weight.
- Tolerate occasional hunger and cravings and learn that you *can* withstand them.
- Make decisions about eating before you encounter triggers. Let's say some friends invite you to dinner. They offer you some tempting dessert. The decision is already made: no. The dessert isn't on your plan, so you don't eat it. You don't have to weigh the pros and cons. You just stick to your plan. This eliminates the tension and struggle.

Plan and monitor your eating in writing every day.

How to Plan

Even if you're following a set meal plan that prescribes what to eat in detail, I still want you to take a few moments now to record your plan for tomorrow. Using your diet notebook, a piece of paper, a note card, your PDA, or your appointment book, write down what you'll eat, how much you'll eat, and when you'll eat it.

Below is a plan that Marcia, one of the dieters I worked with, wrote:

BREAKFAST:
1 banana
1 container nonfat yogurt
1 slice multigrain bread with 1 tablespoon
    reduced-calorie jelly
¼ cup milk (in coffee)

SNACK:
1 piece string cheese
2 whole-wheat crackers

LUNCH:
4 ounces tuna mixed with
    2 tablespoons reduced-
    calorie mayonnaise
1 cup cut-up raw vegetables
    (cherry tomatoes,
    cucumbers, peppers)
3 slices of melon
1 cup skim milk

SNACK:
10 pecans

JUST BEFORE DINNER:
5 to 8 baby carrots

DINNER:
6 ounces cooked chicken with
    3 tablespoons teriyaki sauce
½ medium baked potato with
    2 tablespoons plain yogurt
Salad with lettuce, raw vegetables,
    and 2 tablespoons reduced-fat
    dressing
1 cup broccoli
1 cup green beans with ½ teaspoon
    olive oil
1 apple

SNACK:
1 cup low-fat frozen yogurt
4 cups reduced-fat microwave popcorn

mealtime options

Many people find it easier to sit down for half an hour, create several meal and snack options, and then label them with numbers. Mary wrote down the following options for breakfast:

Breakfast Option 1: 1 cup cereal, 1 cup skim milk, 1 piece of fruit

Breakfast Option 2: 2 scrambled eggs, 1 piece of fruit, 1 low-fat mozzarella cheese stick

Breakfast Option 3: 1 cup low-fat cottage cheese, 1 medium banana

Breakfast Option 4: 1 cup oatmeal, 1 cup skim milk, 1 piece of fruit

She also wrote down several options for snacks, lunches, and dinners. Each evening, Mary chose from these options for the next day. This cut down on her planning time considerably.

Once you've written your plan, make sure you have the food or the ingredients to make the food. Is there anything you can do today to make tomorrow go more smoothly, such as cutting up vegetables for tomorrow's dinner? Make tomorrow's lunch? Now figure out how you're going to keep your written plan with you throughout the day.

Looking Ahead

Tomorrow will be your first official weigh-in. You'll step on the scale first thing in the morning and write your weight in your diet notebook. You'll need to refer to the number next week when you weigh again and create a weight-loss graph to help you monitor your progress (page 174).

Follow these pointers:

- Try to wear same-weight clothing for all your weigh-ins.
- Step on the scale only once. Don't weigh yourself a second time, hoping for a lower weight. It doesn't really matter, and it'll only make you obsessive.
- Don't think of your weight as a catastrophe or criticize yourself. It doesn't matter if you weigh 125, 150, 250, or 350 pounds tomorrow. Whether you have a little or a lot to lose, you're going to use the skills you're learning in this book for your whole life. It doesn't matter if it takes you four weeks or four years to reach your goal. You're going to be doing the same things for a very long time.

what are you thinking?

Does the idea of planning seem unfair, punitive, or too regimented? I can tell you from experience that there just isn't another way. You're right in a certain sense that it's unfair to have to plan. After all, many people who aren't dieting don't have to plan like this. They can stand in front of the refrigerator and think, *What do I feel like eating tonight?* People who want to lose weight, however, just can't have that luxury. Even if you can make good choices now, the time will come (in a few days or weeks) when allowing yourself to make spontaneous decisions will lead to gaining weight.

So, if you think, *I don't* have *to do this part of the program,* acknowledge that the reality is probably, *I don't* want *to do this part of the program.* For just one week, commit to writing down everything you're going to eat the next day. At the end of the week, decide whether to commit to another week. Committing to one week at a time is easier than saying you're going to do this for life—especially since you probably won't need to! Some people find that recording what they eat for a few weeks or months is enough. Can't commit to a full week? Then at least commit to today and tomorrow!

Let's say you give it a try for a day, a week, or many months. How do you know when you can stop? When you find that you're using the tools in this book consistently—and consistently losing weight—stop planning and see what happens. If you can follow your diet conscientiously, that's great. If not, go back to writing and monitoring for a while.

If you're having sabotaging thoughts, get ready to write your Response Cards.

Sabotaging Thought: I don't want to write anything down.
Helpful Response: Which is stronger: wanting to lose weight or not wanting to be inconvenienced? Since I do want to lose weight, I'm going to start writing. It'll probably take only five minutes. I have a choice. I can listen to the resistant part of my mind, or I can firmly and decisively decide to do the writing, even though I feel resistant. It's great practice to ignore my resistant feelings because they'll come up again and again when I don't feel like following my eating plan.

Sabotaging Thought: I can follow a diet without having to do this.
Helpful Response: That might be true—at first—but why not maximize my chances?

Sabotaging Thought: Writing a food plan won't make me lose weight.
Helpful Response: If the program only consisted of writing food plans, it wouldn't work. In this program, however, writing a plan is just one strategy. In any case, I won't know if I'll be successful until I try it. I may as well do everything in my power that I can because I really want to lose weight.

Sabotaging Thought: I'll write it down later.
Helpful Response: I may not get to it later. I have to make this a priority right now.

commit in writing

In order to eliminate spontaneous eating so I can lose weight, I'm going to plan the next day's eating each evening at: _____.

Once I accept the fact that I have to
write a food plan every evening for the
next day, dieting will be easier.

today's to-do list

Check off the tasks you've completed. For any item you haven't completed, record when you're going to complete it.

_____ I read my Advantages Response Card at least twice today.

_____ I read my other Response Cards as needed.

_____ I ate slowly, sitting down and noticing every bite.

Circle one: Every time   Most of the time   Some of the time

_____ I gave myself credit when I engaged in helpful eating behaviors.

Circle one: Every time   Most of the time   Some of the time

_____ I did spontaneous exercise.

Circle one: Every opportunity   Some of the time   Once or twice   Not at all

_____ I did planned exercise.

_____ I tolerated hunger and craving rather than giving in.

_____ I wrote out a food plan for tomorrow.

chapter 7

Week 3

Go: Start Your Diet

It doesn't matter if you're starting a diet for the second time or the twentieth time. The knowledge you've gained and the practice you've put in for the past two weeks make you more equipped than you've ever been to:

- Plan what you're going to eat.
- Eat in a healthy way.
- Resist hunger and cravings.
- Respond to sabotaging thoughts that lead to unplanned eating.
- Give yourself credit and build your confidence that this time you *can* succeed.

These are all life changes that will become a part of your new mindset as you continue to practice your skills every day. Are you surprised by how much you've learned? If you're starting your diet this week (or if you started it a while ago), don't you feel better prepared? For example, you now know two crucially important things about hunger and craving: The first is that you can tolerate these uncomfortable sensations no matter what and that if you don't give in to them then they'll pass. The second is that you can make them pass much faster by using your anti-craving techniques, changing your mindset, and engaging in helpful behaviors. Now, you'll know what to do for the rest of your life.

This week, you'll learn additional Cognitive Therapy techniques to greatly strengthen your resistance muscle and be better able to reject tempting food—even if it's right in front of you. If you struggle with dieting because of the characteristics I described in Chapter 3 (pages 33–43), you'll take big steps this week toward changing your mindset. You'll start to evolve from someone who struggles with dieting to someone who thinks like a thin person.

Give yourself credit and
build your confidence that this time
you *can* succeed.

day 15
Monitor Your Eating

Even if you're already following a diet, don't skip today's task. It's essential! If you're starting your diet today, let me start by congratulating you. Today marks an important change in your life. Give yourself credit for getting this far.

The first thing you're going to do is weigh yourself. If you wear clothes when you weigh yourself, wear about the same weight clothing each morning that you get on the scale. Mark down your weight in your diet notebook. Next, do the following:

Follow your food plan. Eat only what's on the plan you wrote for yourself last night. Eat everything on the plan, unless you become overly full before you've finished, and don't skip a meal.

Monitor your eating immediately after finishing each meal and snack by noting what you ate on your food plan.

Give yourself credit every single time you stick to your plan. Say to yourself, *That's good! I ate what I was supposed to, and I'm taking the time to check it off.*

Respond to sabotaging thoughts if you eat something you shouldn't. If you think, *Why did I eat that? I didn't really even want it ... I'm an idiot,* counter it in a helpful way, such as, *Okay, I ate something I hadn't planned ... It isn't that big a deal ... I can get back on track right this minute, and it's really good that I wrote it down.*

At the end of the day, look at how you marked up your food plan. Give yourself credit for everything you did well. Did you eat anything you hadn't planned? If so, get into problem-solving mode and figure out what you need to do in the future to eliminate this kind of eating. For example, if you get too hungry between meals, perhaps you need to plan heartier meals or to add in a snack. If you eat out of boredom, schedule your time differently. If you need help, call your diet coach.

Follow this sequence every day, for a long time to come.

The Benefits of Writing Down What You Eat

Several studies show that keeping a written record of what you eat increases the likelihood that you'll lose weight and keep it off. One study conducted at St. Francis Medical Center in Peoria, Illinois, found that dieters who kept detailed food logs were even able to lose weight over the winter holiday season. Dieters who didn't keep a log *gained* weight.

Monitoring what you eat in writing as you eat it facilitates your sticking to your diet for the following reasons:

It helps you remain accountable for what you actually eat. You might think you don't have to take the trouble to record what you're eating, that you can just keep a mental tally. Yet, it's truly amazing what our minds both naturally forget and allow us to forget when we don't really want to remember. Even the most nutritionally adept—such as registered dietitians—are guilty of forgetting about some of what they eat. In a study completed at Louisiana State University, researchers asked dietitians to estimate the number of calories they were consuming. The dietitians underreported their actual caloric intake by 10 percent!

We don't necessarily consciously lie to ourselves about what we've eaten. It's just that it's really easy to forget about the small amounts of leftovers, the cream in our coffee, the second helpings at meals, the tastes we're offered in the supermarket. Checking off what you've eaten and writing down what you hadn't planned to eat forces you to become aware of what you're doing. You can't fool yourself when you're looking at the evidence in black and white.

tip! At some point during your diet, I guarantee that you'll feel tempted to stop monitoring in writing what you eat. Usually, this happens when you stray from your diet and are trying to avoid facing it and feeling bad. When you notice this temptation, take a step back. It's 10 times more important to write things down at these times. Beware of the sabotaging thought that says, *It doesn't matter if I don't record my food intake this time.* Of course it matters.

*Checking off what you've eaten and
writing down what you hadn't planned to
eat forces you to become aware of
what you're doing.*

Continually monitoring what you eat will provide you with the following benefits:

It helps you strengthen your motivation. It gives you an opportunity to give yourself credit, especially when you consciously tell yourself how good it is that you ate according to your plan.

It helps you build your confidence. As you focus on how well you're following your plan, you begin to realize that you *can* stay on a diet, that you *can* do what it takes to lose weight.

It helps you recognize and solve problems. By taking time each night to see if you strayed from your eating plan—and why—you can figure out how to correct the problem in the future. Instead of labeling yourself as a failure for overeating or engaging in unplanned eating, you can see these behaviors as solvable problems and not as personal failures.

*Dieters who kept detailed food
logs were even able to lose weight over
the winter holiday season.*

How to Monitor in Writing What You Eat

Carry the food plan you wrote the night before with you throughout the day. As soon as possible after you finish eating, make three kinds of notations:

1. Put a check mark next to the things you ate that were written on your plan.
2. Cross out anything you had planned to eat but didn't.
3. Circle any food that you ate too much of and write down and circle any food you ate that you hadn't planned to eat.

Be sure to make these notations immediately after eating. If you wait, you won't be as conscious of what you're eating, you'll be at higher risk of unplanned eating, and you'll forget about some of the food you ate—all of which increases the risk of your gaining weight.

Below is how Marcia marked up her food plan (see page 136). As you can see, Marcia ate the foods she had planned, except the bread at breakfast and green beans at dinner. For dinner, she also ate an extra half of a baked potato that she hadn't planned, as well as squash. Marcia repeatedly told me that had she not been keeping written records, she definitely would have strayed from her food plan much more often.

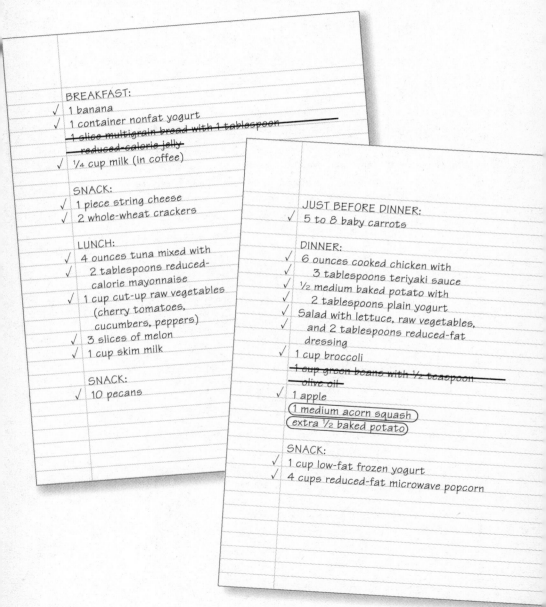

BREAKFAST:
√ 1 banana
√ 1 container nonfat yogurt
~~1 slice multigrain bread with 1 tablespoon reduced-calorie jelly~~
√ ¼ cup milk (in coffee)

SNACK:
√ 1 piece string cheese
√ 2 whole-wheat crackers

LUNCH:
√ 4 ounces tuna mixed with
√ 2 tablespoons reduced-calorie mayonnaise
√ 1 cup cut-up raw vegetables (cherry tomatoes, cucumbers, peppers)
√ 3 slices of melon
√ 1 cup skim milk

SNACK:
√ 10 pecans

JUST BEFORE DINNER:
√ 5 to 8 baby carrots

DINNER:
√ 6 ounces cooked chicken with
√ 3 tablespoons teriyaki sauce
√ ½ medium baked potato with
√ 2 tablespoons plain yogurt
√ Salad with lettuce, raw vegetables,
√ and 2 tablespoons reduced-fat dressing
√ 1 cup broccoli
~~1 cup green beans with ½ teaspoon olive oil~~
√ 1 apple
(1 medium acorn squash)
(extra ½ baked potato)

SNACK:
√ 1 cup low-fat frozen yogurt
√ 4 cups reduced-fat microwave popcorn

Marcia wasn't at all happy initially with the idea of keeping a food plan. She did so half-heartedly for the first week and then not at all during the second week. I asked her about it.

Dr. Beck: So you weren't able to keep your food log at all this week?

Marcia: I don't know, it just seems like so much trouble.

Dr. Beck: How much time does it take to write it down at night?

Marcia: *[thinks]* Uh, I'm not sure.

Dr. Beck: How about if we have you write down tomorrow's food plan right now? Would that be okay?

Marcia: *[reluctantly]* I guess so.

Marcia wrote down her plan. It took her less than three minutes.

Marcia: I'm surprised! I thought I remember it taking, like, 10 or 15 minutes.

Dr. Beck: So it wasn't as much trouble as you thought?

Marcia: No, I guess not.

Dr. Beck: And, tomorrow, how long will it take to check off what you actually ate after breakfast?

Marcia: A couple of seconds, I guess.

Dr. Beck: Would it be the same for your snacks and other meals?

Marcia: Yeah.

Dr. Beck: Okay, let's imagine it's tomorrow night. You're thinking, *I guess I'd better write down my food plan for tomorrow.* How are you feeling?

Marcia: *[sighs]* A little resistant, I think.

Dr. Beck: What's going through your mind?

Marcia: I don't really want to do this.

Dr. Beck: What else are you thinking?

Marcia: I'm tired. I don't have the energy. Besides, maybe I don't really need it. I know what I'm supposed to eat.

Dr. Beck: Okay. Do you have your Advantages Response Card with you? Can you pull it out and read it to me right now?

Marcia pulls out the card and reads it aloud.

Dr. Beck: How important are these things to you?

Marcia: Pretty important.

Dr. Beck: What seems more important to you: being able to skip writing down your food plan or being able to look better, to feel better, to be more attractive, to be less self-conscious ...

Marcia: *[interrupts]* The advantages are more important.

Dr. Beck: Are you sure?

Marcia: Yeah, I'm sure *[pauses]* but …

Dr. Beck: But?

Marcia: But I wish I didn't have to write down my plan.

Dr. Beck: Do you remember what we talked about over the past couple of weeks— about *why* you need to write down your plan? After all, you've lost some weight. So why do it?

Marcia: Well, you said that dieting would be easier for the first couple of weeks but that there would come a time when my motivation would probably go down.

Dr. Beck: Exactly. And then what would happen?

Marcia: I guess what's happened all those other times I tried to diet. I'd start eating what I wasn't supposed to and then give it all up.

Dr. Beck: So we already know what *doesn't* work. It *doesn't* work to just decide at the last minute what you're going to eat. Because, when your motivation is lower, you'll eat foods that aren't on your diet.

Marcia: Yeah.

Dr. Beck: But if you're already in the habit of writing down a plan every night and checking it off every day…?

Marcia: I guess it could help.

Dr. Beck: Do you think you'd say to yourself, *No, don't eat it, or you'll have to write it down?*

Marcia: Yeah, probably.

Dr. Beck: And that would help you resist?

Marcia: I think it would.

Dr. Beck: Now, how bad does it seem to write down your plan for three minutes every night, when you realize that it *will* help you be thinner, feel more attractive, feel better about yourself …

Marcia: It's not so bad. I'm not sure why I was so resistant.

Dr. Beck: Well, it's because you had those sabotaging thoughts. But now you know how to answer them back. How about if you write down your answers on a Response Card now so that you can read it every night, right after dinner, along with your Advantages Response Card?

Marcia: Okay.

Marcia made the following Response Card:

> If I start to resist writing down my plan tonight, I'll remind myself:
>
> * I'm going to need it when my motivation goes down.
> * I haven't been able to stick to a diet without doing it.
> * It'll take only three minutes at most.
> * I really want to lose weight because of all the advantages.

what are you thinking?

While research has consistently shown the importance of keeping written food records, many studies also show that few dieters keep them. One study even found that fewer than a third of dieters wrote down all of the foods they ate on just half of the days they were supposed to keep records! I'll bet these participants had lots of sabotaging thoughts that got in the way.

Use the following examples to create Response Cards that will increase the likelihood that you'll consistently keep your written food record every day.

Sabotaging Thought: This is too much work.
Helpful Response: I won't have to write things down for the rest of my life. Besides, it'll probably be less burdensome than I'm predicting. Why not give the "best" option a try for a week and see how it goes?

Sabotaging Thought: I don't need to write this down; I can remember what I ate.
Helpful Response: Not writing things down hasn't helped me in the past. I undoubtedly forget about some of the food that I eat. I have to make myself conscious of what I'm eating.

Sabotaging Thought: I'll wait until I've lost some weight. Then I'll feel more motivated to do this task.
Helpful Response: If I wait, chances are excellent that I'll never do it.

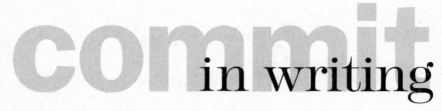

commit in writing

I'll make written notations about exactly what I ate: _____

_____. (I hope you wrote, "immediately after I've finished eating.")

Once I accept the fact that I have to monitor
my eating in this way, dieting will be easier.

today's to-do list

It's time to follow up on how you've been doing on your previous tasks. Have you completed all the tasks in Weeks 1 and 2 that prepare you for dieting?

- Have you chosen two diets (a primary and a backup)?
- Have you created time in your schedule and prepared your house and work environments?
- Are you consulting your diet coach regularly?

If not, add these tasks to your to-do list today in addition to checking off the following items. For any item you haven't completed, record when you're going to complete it.

_____ I read my Advantages Response Card at least twice today.

_____ I read other Response Cards as needed.

_____ I ate slowly, sitting down and noticing every bite.

Circle one: Every time   Most of the time   Some of the time

_____ I gave myself credit for engaging in helpful eating behaviors.

Circle one: Every time   Most of the time   Some of the time

_____ I did spontaneous exercise.

Circle one: Every opportunity   Some of the time   Once or twice   Not at all

_____ I did planned exercise.

_____ I monitored everything that I ate today in writing right after I ate it.

_____ I wrote out a new food plan for tomorrow.

_____ I weighed myself and recorded my weight.

day 16
Prevent Unplanned Eating

Some people don't struggle much when they're deciding when and what to eat. They just open the cabinet or refrigerator and select what they want. If you're like most dieters, though, you've struggled at times when you were tempted to eat something you shouldn't. You probably had a dialogue in your mind that went something like this: *I really want to eat this. But I know I shouldn't. But I really want it. I'm not supposed to have it. But I feel like having it! I know it's not on my food plan, but I don't care. I'm going to have it anyway.*

This internal argument can create tension, which is emotionally and physically uncomfortable. You'll be tempted to relieve this tension by eating. Once you make the decision to eat, you may find that your discomfort immediately subsides—even *before* you reach for the food. You can do other things, though, to reduce your discomfort. Just as deciding to eat can reduce tension, so can deciding *not* to eat.

Your written food plan will help you make your decision ahead of time—*before* you're confronted with uncomfortable cravings and tension. But it won't eliminate indecision. There will be times when you begin to argue with yourself. Perhaps you're at a party and want a glass of wine that's not on your plan. Perhaps a coworker asks you to try a brownie she baked. The triggers for eating are endless, but the solution is straightforward: *Tell yourself that you don't have a choice. You made a plan, and you'll follow that plan—no ifs, ands, or buts.*

Firmly saying, *NO CHOICE*, decreases both the struggle and the discomfort. Think about rules you already have in your life. Do you struggle over whether or not to brush your teeth? Imagine how annoying it would be if you had to fight to get yourself to do this mundane task everyday! But you don't struggle because you have a rule: *I have to brush every day.*

You also might establish other "no choice" rules. I've made some eating rules for myself that I rarely break. I don't even think much about it; I just follow them. I don't struggle, I don't feel conflicted, I don't feel deprived, and I don't end up eating food I'll be sorry about moments later.

You made a plan, and you'll follow
that plan—no ifs, ands, or buts.

Following a rule eliminates the struggle over what to eat or not eat.

Here are my rules:

1. Eat a substantial amount of protein, vegetables, and fruit at every meal.

2. Don't eat any junk food until after dinner.

3. Eat only raw vegetables while preparing dinner.

4. When eating out, eat up to only 25 percent more than I usually do when I'm home.

These rules enable me to leave afternoon receptions feeling good and looking forward to dinner. They keep me from gaining more than a couple of pounds when I'm on vacation. Following a rule eliminates the struggle over what to eat or not to eat.

Make a NO CHOICE Response Card

Think about some eating rules that you'd like to establish. You don't need to come up with all of them today. These rules might come to you over time. There is one rule, however, that you have to commit to (you don't have a choice in the matter): You *must* follow your food plan.

To strengthen this idea, make a Response Card similar to the one below. Read this NO CHOICE Response Card at least twice a day and whenever you find yourself struggling over whether or not to eat something.

NO CHOICE

what are you thinking?

If you're having sabotaging thoughts about the necessity of giving up spontaneous eating, prepare Response Cards.

Sabotaging Thought: I deserve to be able to eat what I want.

Helpful Response: If I want all the benefits of being thinner, I just can't eat whatever I want without planning. I have to make "I deserve to be thinner and feel good about myself" a much higher priority than "I deserve to make spontaneous choices about what I eat."

Sabotaging Thought: I don't think that I can accept the fact that I can't eat spontaneously.

Helpful Response: I've been giving myself choices about what, when, and how much to eat for a long time, so it feels natural and right to do so. On the other hand, I have to face the fact that spontaneous eating doesn't work for me. The more often I say, *NO CHOICE,* to myself, the less I'll struggle.

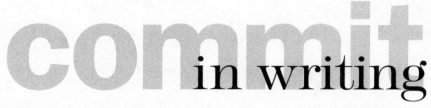

commit in writing

When I feel like eating in an unplanned way, I'll: _____

_____

_____

_____

_____ .

Once I accept the fact that I
have to give up spontaneous eating,
dieting will be easier.

today's to-do list

Check off the tasks you've completed. For any item you haven't completed, record when you're going to complete it.

_____ I read my Advantages Response Card at least twice today.

_____ I read other Response Cards as needed.

_____ I ate slowly, sitting down and noticing every bite.

Circle one: Every time   Most of the time   Some of the time

_____ I gave myself credit for engaging in helpful eating behaviors.

Circle one: Every time   Most of the time   Some of the time

_____ I did spontaneous exercise.

Circle one: Every opportunity   Some of the time   Once or twice   Not at all

_____ I did planned exercise.

_____ I wrote out a food plan for tomorrow.

_____ I monitored everything I ate in writing.

_____ I made my NO CHOICE Response Card.

day 17
End Overeating

Even if you're not tempted to overeat today, you'll undoubtedly face trigger situations many times in the future. If you regularly eat family-style, for example, it might be difficult for you to avoid reaching for seconds. When you're in a restaurant, you're usually served a larger quantity of food than your diet plan allows and you might be tempted to clean your plate. Today, you'll practice not overeating.

There are two circumstances you might face while dieting that qualify as overeating:

- **If you eat any food in a greater quantity than you had planned.** Maybe you had written down last night that you were going to eat 6 ounces of chicken but instead you ate 10 ounces. Or maybe you had planned to eat 1 cup of vegetables, but since your diet plan allows you to have an unlimited amount of them, you ended up eating 2 cups.
- **If you feel full partway through your meal** but continue to finish it anyway, leading to a feeling of overfullness.

In order for you to successfully lose weight and keep it off, you must know how to identify when you're no longer hungry so that you can stop eating.

Overload Your Plate—and Don't Eat It All

Today, you'll practice *not* overeating by purposely putting more food on your plate than you plan to eat. Pick one meal, preferably lunch or dinner. Choose a food that's on your plan, but then I want you to purposely give yourself a larger portion than you would normally allow. Also, choose a food that you're not supposed to eat and put it on your plate. At the beginning of the meal, push the extra portions to the side on your plate. Then eat only the food on your plan.

If you're tempted to eat the extra food, use some of the anti-craving techniques you learned on Day 13 (pages 127–134). If you find that you still want to eat what's left on your plate, counter your sabotaging thoughts. For example, if you think, *It's a shame that I can't eat this … It's bad to waste food,* then tell yourself, *Isn't it great that I'm not eating this … This is getting me closer to my goal of losing weight … This is helping me to strengthen my resistance muscle.*

Also remind yourself just how good you'll feel if you *don't* overeat versus how bad you'll feel if you *do*. Look back and reflect on the consequences of overeating in the past. Are you glad that you overate then, given that it contributed to your current weight? Or are you sorry? Is the ratio of being sorry to glad now about 20,000 to 1? Ask yourself, *How glad will I be in 10 minutes if I overeat now?*

When you've finished eating just the food you're supposed to eat, clear your plate. Throw out the extra food or save it for another meal. If it was easy to do this task, you might never need to repeat it. On the other hand, if you found it difficult to resist eating the extra food, don't despair. Give yourself credit for trying and see what you can learn from the experience. Then repeat this exercise until it gets easy.

For the rest of your life, expect to encounter many situations in which you don't have control over the food you're served (at restaurants, events, and friends'/families' houses) when you'll benefit from this kind of practice. You may find it especially helpful to try this exercise again the day before you know you'll be entering a situation in which you'll be tempted to overeat.

> In order to successfully lose
> weight and keep it off, *you have to stop eating
> when you've eaten the amount
> of food on your plan.*

in session with Dr. Beck

When I asked Angela to do this overeating exercise, she thought it would be easy. She was very surprised when she found out how hard it was. She told me about her experience at our next session.

Dr. Beck: So, Angela, did you try the experiment? Did you put extra food on your plate?
Angela: *[takes a deep breath]* Yeah, I tried it yesterday.
Dr. Beck: How did it go?
Angela: It was hard—really hard!
Dr. Beck: Tell me what happened.

Angela: At dinner last night I put extra chicken on my plate—almost a whole portion extra.

Dr. Beck: And then?

Angela: I don't know. It made me really nervous.

Dr. Beck: What were you thinking?

Angela: I ... I just didn't like having it on there. I didn't like the idea of having food on my plate that I couldn't eat.

Dr. Beck: What did you think could happen?

Angela: I was afraid I'd just go ahead and eat it.

Dr. Beck: Did you?

Angela: No, but I ended up getting up halfway through dinner and putting the extra chicken in the refrigerator.

Dr. Beck: So you were able to do half the experiment.

Angela: Yeah.

Dr. Beck: When you had the thought, *I might go ahead and eat it,* did you answer that thought back?

Angela: I'm not sure what you mean.

Dr. Beck: Did you say to yourself, *If I want to eat it, I can stop myself by using anti-craving techniques?* Did you remember that you could use them?

Angela: No, I guess it didn't even cross my mind.

Dr. Beck: Can you think about it now? What anti-craving techniques could you have tried if you were tempted to eat the extra chicken?

Angela: I guess I could have just left the table and done something for a few minutes and then come back.

Dr. Beck: Right! What do you think might have happened if you'd responded to your sabotaging thought by saying to yourself, *If I'm tempted, I can always get up and distract myself.* Would you have felt as nervous?

Angela: No, I don't think so.

Dr. Beck: Do you think you could have gotten through the meal without eating it?

Angela: Yeah, probably.

Dr. Beck: Okay, so how about trying this experiment again? Could you do it at lunch or dinner tonight?

Angela: Yeah, I'll try it.

Dr. Beck: Do you think it would be better if you tried it first with an easier food? Is there something else you've planned to eat that you definitely would feel more comfortable leaving on your plate?

Angela: Yeah. I'm having steamed green beans tonight, leftover from the other day. I could put a bunch of extra ones on my plate.

Dr. Beck: Okay, start with that. Then maybe tomorrow you could put just a small amount of extra chicken on your plate. And the next day, a slightly larger piece, so you can build up your confidence. Does that sound okay?

Angela: Yeah, I'll try that.

Dr. Beck: Now, if you have any trouble, it'll be because of your sabotaging thoughts. Let's have you make a Response Card right now.

Angela made the following Response Card:

> When I feel anxious about having extra food on my plate, I'll remind myself that even if I want to eat it, I can use anti-craving techniques.

what are you thinking?

Notice your thoughts. What sabotaging thoughts are getting in the way of completing this experiment? Here are some common ones along with helpful responses.

Sabotaging Thought: I don't need to do this. I'll be able to stop eating without practicing this skill.

Helpful Response: This isn't a big deal. I should try it anyway. The worst thing that could happen is that I didn't need to do it. I might not learn from this, but I also might learn a lot.

Sabotaging Thought: I hate to deliberately waste food.

Helpful Response: Which is better: deliberately wasting food or overeating and gaining weight? What would I tell my best friend if she had this problem? The truth is that the extra food will either go to waste in my body or go to waste in the garbage. Either way, it'll go to waste. And no matter what I heard from my parents when I was growing up, overeating doesn't help starving people any place in the world.

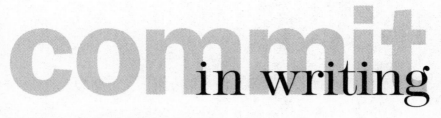

commit in writing

To learn the skill of not overeating, I'm going to: _____
_____
_____
_____
_____.

> Once I learn to stop eating even
> though there's still food on my plate,
> dieting will be easier.

today's to-do list

Check off the tasks you've completed. For any item you haven't completed, record when you're going to complete it.

_____ I read my Advantages and NO CHOICE Response Cards at least twice today.

_____ I read my other Response Cards as needed.

_____ I ate slowly, sitting down and noticing every bite.

          Circle one: Every time   Most of the time   Some of the time

_____ I gave myself credit for engaging in helpful eating behaviors.

          Circle one: Every time   Most of the time   Some of the time

_____ I did spontaneous exercise.

          Circle one: Every opportunity   Some of the time   Once or twice   Not at all

_____ I did planned exercise.

_____ I wrote out a food plan for tomorrow.

_____ I monitored everything I ate in writing right after I finished eating.

_____ I practiced not overeating.

day 18

Change Your Definition of Full

Since the beginning of this week, you've been planning what you're going to eat before you eat it. Do you wonder, *Why can't I just eat when I'm hungry and stop eating once I'm full?*

Ideally, you *would* eat only when you're hungry and stop eating when you're almost full or mildly full. Chances are, however, that you're not naturally good at this skill. Most of the dieters I've counseled didn't know how to recognize when they were really hungry and when they weren't. When they relied on hunger signals to guide their eating, they invariably overate.

Here's a way to determine if you've overeaten: Think about how easy it would be to take a walk at a moderate to brisk pace before you eat. You should be able to walk at the same pace just as easily *after* a meal, too. If you can't easily take a moderate to brisk walk after a meal, it means that you've eaten too much and you might have an unrealistic definition of fullness.

People without weight problems feel somewhat uncomfortable when they eat to the point where they can't comfortably take a walk after a meal. But when you eat to that point, you might not feel the same discomfort. The sensations you notice might feel normal to you. Your definition of fullness might be part of the reason you gained weight in the first place or have had difficulty losing weight.

You might eat beyond the point of normal fullness for several other reasons, too: One, you might want to prolong the eating experience—that is, have food in your mouth for a longer period of time. Two, you might have difficulty turning your attention away from eating if you know there's food readily available. Three, you might be concerned that if you don't load up now, you'll be too hungry before you can have your next meal or snack. You might link the sensation of overfullness with feeling safe or protected from discomfort. In other words, you eat more now to avoid feeling hungry later.

> If you can't easily take a moderate to brisk walk after a meal, it means you've eaten too much and *you might have an unrealistic definition of fullness.*

Break the Connection

In order to lose excess weight and keep it off, you must break the connection between overfullness and normal fullness. To do so, you'll need lots and lots of experiences of eating to normal fullness and saying to yourself, *This is great that I'm stopping now.* You'll then begin to associate overfullness with feeling abnormal. Once you change the connection, you'll struggle so much less and feel so much less deprived. Do the following:

- For a month, after each meal, ask yourself, *Could I easily go for a moderate to brisk walk?* If you're not sure whether or not you can, try it.

- If the answer is yes, tell yourself, *Good, then I'm experiencing normal fullness.*

- If the answer is no, tell yourself, *This is what overfullness feels like ... It's not normal ... At my next meal, I'm going to make sure I don't put too much food on my plate.*

- Every time you'd like to overeat but don't, give yourself credit. You might say, for example, *It's great that I'm exercising my resistance muscle.*

- If you're triggered to overeat, remove the triggers. For example, if you're serving yourself a family-style meal, move the serving dishes to the side of the table away from you after everyone has taken portions. If someone serves you too much food, move the extra amounts to the side of your plate. Get another family member to put away leftovers, as well as clear and scrape the dishes.

- Respond to your sabotaging thoughts. When you've finished what you planned to eat, you might think, *Oh, I really want to eat more.* If so, tell yourself, *No, I'm normally full ... I want to be thinner, so I'm going to stop eating now.*

- If you feel anxious, remind yourself that hunger is not an emergency. Remember, you *can* tolerate the feeling—you proved this to yourself on Day 12 (pages 121–126). Hunger will come and go, and you certainly *can* wait to eat until your next scheduled snack or meal—there's always another coming.

tip! If you finish what's on your plate and feel disappointed that you can't eat more, remind yourself that you'll be able to eat again soon. You might say, *It's okay, I'm going to have a snack in three hours—an apple and a cheese stick ... I can wait.* Then immediately read your Advantages Response Card to remind yourself why it's worth putting up with this momentary disappointment.

If you easily stop eating before you're overly full, you might only need to practice today's task once. On the other hand, if you struggle to stop eating before you've overeaten, you might need to continually work on this skill for several weeks.

what are you thinking?

Are you feeling resistant about recognizing that you have to eat less? Then read the following sabotaging thoughts and create Response Cards based on the responses below.

Sabotaging Thought: I like feeling really, really full.
Helpful Response: I need to accept that this sensation is not what is considered normal. I'm really eating beyond fullness, which has contributed to my being overweight.

Sabotaging Thought: My diet plan says I'm allowed to have unlimited amounts of certain foods. What's the harm of eating lots of them?
Helpful Response: I'm going to have many, many experiences in which I don't have access to these unlimited foods: at restaurants, buffets, and social gatherings. If I haven't repeatedly practiced eating to normal fullness, I'm likely to eat too much of the foods I have to limit in those situations.

Sabotaging Thought: What if I end up feeling hungry before it's time to eat again?
Helpful Response: I learned on Day 12 that hunger is not an emergency, that I can tolerate the sensations of hunger, and that, if I don't focus on it, the hunger *will* dissipate. If I still don't feel confident in my abilities to tolerate hunger, I should repeat the Day 12 tasks (pages 121–126) in addition to completing today's task.

commit in writing

When I recognize that I'm probably normally full, I'm going to: _____
_____
_____
_____
_____
_____.

Once I change my definition of fullness, dieting will be easier.

today's to-do list

Check off the tasks you've completed. For any item you haven't completed, record when you're going to complete it.

_____ I read my Advantages and NO CHOICE Response Cards at least twice today.

_____ I read my other Response Cards as needed.

_____ I ate slowly, sitting down and noticing every bite.

Circle one: Every time   Most of the time   Some of the time

_____ I gave myself credit for engaging in helpful eating behaviors.

Circle one: Every time   Most of the time   Some of the time

_____ I did spontaneous exercise.

Circle one: Every opportunity   Some of the time   Once or twice   Not at all

_____ I did planned exercise.

_____ I wrote out a food plan for tomorrow.

_____ I monitored everything I ate in writing right after I finished eating.

_____ I ate only to normal fullness.

Circle one: Every time   Most of the time   Some of the time

day 19

Stop Fooling Yourself

Dieters have an amazing ability to delude themselves about food. They might be very rational and reasonable in other ways, but not when it comes to dieting. Think about times you've dieted and were supposed to limit what you ate. Did you give yourself a "fake" excuse to eat?

Read the following list of self-deluding sabotaging thoughts and check off those that you've had in the past.

It's okay to eat this because ...

- ○ it's not a whole piece.
- ○ I'll eat it only this one time.
- ○ it's not that fattening.
- ○ I'll make up for it by eating less later.
- ○ it won't matter.
- ○ I paid for it.
- ○ it'll go to waste.
- ○ I'll disappoint someone if I don't.
- ○ everyone else is eating it.
- ○ I'm celebrating.
- ○ no one will see me eating it.
- ○ it's just the crumbs.
- ○ it's free.
- ○ I really want it.
- ○ it's a special occasion.
- ○ I'm upset, and I just don't care.
- ○ I'm craving it, and I'll probably just eat it eventually.

These thoughts delude you into eating when you shouldn't. After all, a calorie is a calorie, no matter when, where, or why you eat it. You might be able to see how irrational these thoughts are right now. Yet, in the moment when you really want to eat something, you might try to convince yourself that these thoughts are valid.

How to Stop Fooling Yourself

The next time you have an urge to eat something that's not on your plan, notice what's going through your mind. Only on rare occasions do people put food in their mouths without thinking about it. There's usually a thought that

measuring up

If your diet calls for you to measure the quantity of food you're supposed to eat, don't fool yourself into thinking you can accurately estimate it instead. Dieters who don't measure or weigh their food are notorious for underestimating their portions. It might not matter much right now if you eat a little extra at every meal because you didn't measure, but at some point it will. You need to squarely face your food decisions. If you're going to eat more food than your diet program calls for, do so because you've deliberately planned to, not because you've falsely reassured yourself, *It's okay if I don't really know how much I'm eating.*

You won't have to measure food for the rest of your life, however. As soon as you become adept at visualizing portion sizes, you can stop. (Of course, whenever you introduce a new food into your diet, you'll need to measure it.)

How will you know when you're ready to stop measuring? Serve yourself food and then measure it before you eat. If you're quite close, you're probably ready to stop measuring those foods. It's a good idea to measure your food periodically, though, to make sure you're still estimating portion sizes accurately.

precedes eating. Pay particular attention to thoughts that start with the phrase, *It's okay to eat this because….*

These are usually fooling-yourself thoughts. You need to prepare yourself in advance for these kinds of thoughts. Create an It's Not Okay Response Card similar to the one below and read it daily, perhaps whenever you read your Advantages Response Card. Also, pull it out whenever you think you're at risk of not following your plan.

It's Not Okay

It's not okay to eat unplanned food of any kind. I'm just trying to fool myself. Every single time I eat something I'm not supposed to, I strengthen my giving-in muscle and weaken my resistance muscle. I might feel good for the few seconds I'm eating, but I'll feel bad afterwards. If I want to lose excess weight and keep it off, I absolutely must stop fooling myself.

what are you thinking?

You might not have many self-deluding, sabotaging thoughts right this minute. But these thoughts probably will surface later, when you want to eat something you shouldn't. Be prepared and have your responses ready.

Sabotaging Thought: It's okay to eat this because the amount of food is so small.
Helpful Response: Just because it doesn't have many calories doesn't mean I should eat it. I shouldn't! I need to use every opportunity I can to break myself of the habit of eating things I haven't planned.

Sabotaging Thought: It's okay to eat this because otherwise I'm wasting money.
Helpful Response: I'm better off wasting money than gaining weight.

Sabotaging Thought: It's okay to eat this because everyone else is eating it.
Helpful Response: I have to decide whether I want to eat like everyone else and remain overweight or control my eating and lose weight.

Sabotaging Thought: It's okay to eat this because I want it—and, besides, I don't really care!
Helpful Response: I might not care right at this moment, but I'll care in a few minutes—I'll be very unhappy if I eat something I shouldn't. And I sure will care when I find that I'm not losing weight!

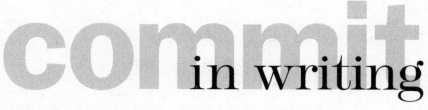

commit in writing

The next time I catch myself thinking a self-deluding thought, I'm going to: _____

_____

_____

_____

_____

_____ .

> Once I stop fooling myself about my
> eating, dieting will be easier.

today's to-do list

Check off the tasks you've completed. For any item you haven't completed, record when you're going to complete it.

_____ I read my Advantages and NO CHOICE Response Cards at least twice today.

_____ I read other Response Cards as needed.

_____ I ate slowly, sitting down and noticing every bite.

Circle one: Every time   Most of the time   Some of the time

_____ I gave myself credit for engaging in helpful eating behaviors.

Circle one: Every time   Most of the time   Some of the time

_____ I did spontaneous exercise.

Circle one: Every opportunity   Some of the time   Once or twice   Not at all

_____ I did planned exercise.

_____ I wrote out a food plan for tomorrow.

_____ I monitored everything I ate in writing right after I finished eating.

_____ I ate only to normal fullness.

_____ I created an It's Not Okay Response Card.

day 20

Get Back on Track

Yesterday, you learned about fooling-yourself thoughts that tend to talk you into giving in to desires and cravings. Today, you'll learn how to respond to a specific fooling-yourself thought—the one that encourages you to abandon your diet *for the whole day* after you've eaten something you weren't supposed to. Your thinking might go like this, *I can't believe I let myself eat this! I've really blown it ... I might as well eat whatever I want for the rest of the day and start dieting again tomorrow.*

But there's no reason to wait. Have you really blown it completely? Of course not!

What did you eat? An extra hamburger? A doughnut? A slice of pie? Let's say you ate some food that contained 500 calories. To gain 1 pound, you have to eat in the neighborhood of 3,500 extra calories—seven times what you ate. An extra 500 calories is *not* going to noticeably affect your weight. So you've eaten 500 extra calories—so what? Does it make more sense to stop now or to keep eating? There's no reason to keep eating and take in an extra 100, 200, 300, or even 3,000 calories.

This idea is shown graphically on the facing page. See what happens when you try to fool yourself? Of course, it's better to stop eating as soon as possible. It's destructive to continue to eat in an unplanned way for the rest of the day just because you ate something that wasn't on your food plan.

Get Back on Your Diet *Now*

If you're tempted to keep on eating when you know you shouldn't, do the following:

Acknowledge your initial slip. Tell yourself, *Okay, I shouldn't have eaten that ... I made a mistake ... This one mistake is certainly not going to make me gain weight this week.*

Recommit yourself to your diet. Read this chapter again, as well as other parts of the book or relevant Response Cards.

Draw a symbolic line. Don't give yourself until tomorrow to get back on track. Instead say, *Here's the line, right here, where I stop this unplanned eating.* Mark this line by brushing your teeth, polishing your nails, going out for a walk, calling a friend or your diet coach, or engaging in some other non-eating-related activity.

Large piece of frosted cake
500 calories

Large piece of frosted cake and a doughnut
800 calories

Large piece of frosted cake, a doughnut,
and a dish of ice cream
1,200 calories

Large piece of frosted cake, a doughnut, a dish of ice cream,
and a candy bar
1,500 calories

Large piece of frosted cake, a doughnut, a dish of ice cream,
a candy bar, and a bag of potato chips
2,000 calories

Large piece of frosted cake, a doughnut, a dish of ice cream, a candy bar,
a bag of potato chips, and 3 pieces of cheese
2,300 calories

Large piece of frosted cake, a doughnut, a dish of ice cream, a candy bar,
a bag of potato chips, 3 pieces of cheese, 2 chocolate chip cookies,
a large muffin, 3 tablespoons of peanut butter, and a soft pretzel
3,500 calories

*It's destructive to continue to eat in
an unplanned way for the rest of the day
just because you ate something that
wasn't on your food plan.*

Give yourself credit for stopping—at any point. If you want to keep eating but you don't, you deserve credit! It's important not to let yourself become demoralized. You need to give yourself some slack for being human and making a mistake.

Watch out for feelings of failure and helplessness. When you slip, you might start to feel like a failure and believe that you just can't diet successfully. It's essential to remind yourself that mistakes are inevitable; it's *normal* to stray from your diet from time to time. No one's perfect.

Continue to eat normally. Some people think, *Now that I ate something I wasn't supposed to, I have to make up for it and not eat for the rest of the day.*

If you allow yourself to think this way, you might end up feeling unhappy and resentful or anxious that you'll be too hungry later on. You might then decide to eat everything you want. You need to put this mistake in perspective. It's just not that big a deal. Go ahead and continue with your eating plan for the rest of the day.

Learn from your mistake. Review your mistake with your diet coach. Use this experience as an opportunity for learning, so you can try to limit similar occurrences in the future. For example, did you:

- Forget to review your Advantages, NO CHOICE, and It's Not Okay Response Cards?
- Neglect to plan your food?
- Forget (or not bother) to have your planned food available?
- Meet up with someone who pushed food on you?
- Try to eat like the other people you were with?
- Encounter an unexpected trigger?
- Wind up surrounded by food you hadn't planned to eat?

Jan had certainly not planned to eat a piece of pizza an hour before dinner. But the pizza box was staring her in the face when she opened the refrigerator door to get something to drink. After she ate it (standing up in front of the refrigerator), she realized that she either should have thrown away the leftover pizza or made sure it was wrapped up and placed in the back of the refrigerator. She realized, too, that she had been pretty stressed out when she got home from work and probably should have sat in her car and done some relaxing breathing for at least a couple of minutes before she went into the house.

what is a binge?

Bingeing is an extreme form of overeating. When people binge, they feel a desperate urge to keep eating. They block out their voice of reason and feel out of control, sometimes as if they're almost in a trance. They eat an abnormally large amount of food—often quickly—and become uncomfortably full. Many people have been able to get control over their bingeing by using the techniques in this book. If you've been following this program faithfully but still experience frequent binges, you might need to consult a mental-health professional.

In order to prepare yourself for occasions when you eat something you're not supposed to, create a Get Back on Track Response Card right now. Read it at least once a day, then pull it out and read it again when you need it. Model it after this card:

Get Back on Track

If I've eaten something I shouldn't, I haven't blown it. It's not the end of the world. I can start following my plan again right this minute. Just because I made a mistake doesn't mean I should keep on eating. That makes no sense. It's a million times better to stop now than to allow myself to eat more.

---

what are you thinking?

You might not have the following sabotaging thoughts today, but you probably will have them at some point when you stray from your plan. Add whatever you find useful to your Get Back on Track Response Card.

Sabotaging Thought: I can't believe I ate that! I'll never lose weight!
Helpful Response: What would my diet coach tell me if she knew I ate this? She would say, "Don't feel bad. Everyone overeats from time to time. You can start again right now. It's not such a big deal. Give yourself a break."

Sabotaging Thought: This is too hard. I can't do it. I'll never be able to stop myself from eating like this. I may as well give up.
Helpful Response: Okay, so I made a mistake. This was inevitable. It's unreasonable to expect myself to be perfect every single time. I'm not a failure. I can learn something from this experience to help me the next time.

commit in writing

When I make a mistake and eat something I'm not supposed to, I'm going to: _____
_____
_____ .

Once I regard my slips as just
mistakes and decide to recommit to my plan
immediately, dieting will be easier.

today's to-do list

Check off the tasks you've completed. For any item you haven't completed, record
when you're going to complete it.

_____ I read my Advantages, NO CHOICE, and It's Not Okay Response Cards
at least twice today.

_____ I read other Response Cards as needed.

_____ I ate slowly, sitting down and noticing every bite.

Circle one: Every time   Most of the time   Some of the time

_____ I gave myself credit for engaging in helpful eating behaviors.

Circle one: Every time   Most of the time   Some of the time

_____ I did spontaneous exercise.

Circle one: Every opportunity   Some of the time   Once or twice   Not at all

_____ I did planned exercise.

_____ I wrote out a food plan for tomorrow.

_____ I monitored everything I ate in writing right after I finished eating.

_____ I ate only to normal fullness.

_____ I identified and responded to a self-deluding thought.

_____ I created a Get Back on Track Response Card.

day 21

Get Ready to Weigh In

Tomorrow, you'll step on the scale and find out if you lost weight this week. Weighing yourself is essential. These weekly weigh-ins can help you in the following ways:

They allow you to celebrate and build up your confidence when you've lost weight. It's important for you to recognize how your hard work has directly led to your weight loss (it didn't happen by magic!) and to feel good about these results.

They keep you honest if you've gained weight. If you haven't been following all the steps in the program, regular weigh-ins make you face that you can't get away with doing only the parts of the program you feel like doing.

They help you stay committed to the program. If you're happy with your weight loss, you'll feel motivated to continue doing what you've been doing. If you're disappointed, you can declare that you're going to figure out where you went wrong, reread parts of this book, and start fresh.

But be careful: Weighing yourself can erode your motivation more than it helps *if you step on the scale with the wrong mindset.*

The Numbers on the Scale

Think about previous times when you've weighed yourself and felt unhappy. Does the following scenario seem familiar?

Situation: The scale shows a higher weight than you'd hoped to see.
↓
Sabotaging Thought: *I can't believe it. This is really terrible.*
↓
Emotion: Upset (angry, sad, demoralized, hopeless)
↓
Behavior: Embark on a "bad eating day"

If you view your weight as an indication of how weak, inadequate, or out of control you are, then weight gains (or smaller-than-expected weight losses) can easily result in overeating.

It's important for you to start using the scale as an information tool that provides data you can use to guide your eating. If you took your temperature, you would use the number on the thermometer as a guide to decide whether you should go to work, whether you should take over-the-counter medication, or whether you should call your doctor. When you weigh yourself, use the number on the scale as a guide to decide whether you should keep doing what you're doing or make some changes.

On any given day, *the number on the scale is exactly what it should be,* given what you ate, how much energy you expended in the past few days, the amount of fluid your body is retaining, and other biological influences.

Before you step on the scale, try not to think, *I hope I weigh _____ pounds.* Instead, think, *Last week, I weighed _____ ... Today, I should probably weigh somewhere between a half pound to 2 pounds more or less than that.*

If the number on the scale doesn't go down—or doesn't go down much—and you suspect you've been eating too much, don't waste time blaming yourself and having negative thoughts. Consider what you might be doing wrong and do something positive to solve the problem. Maybe you've become lax about measuring food or counting calories or carbohydrates. Maybe you need to add a few more minutes of planned exercise each day. Ask your diet coach for help in implementing any tasks you need to practice.

If the scale doesn't go down and you know you've been following your diet and exercise plans faithfully, don't panic. You can easily go up or down 2 pounds on any given day due to hormonal or other physiological reasons. If so, you'll undoubtedly lose weight next week if you continue to follow your plan.

q: Can I weigh myself more often than once a week?

a: Yes, and some find that weighing themselves daily helps desensitize them to the scale. Do not, however, weigh yourself more than once a day. Doing so is a sure sign that you're obsessing about dieting and not keeping a healthy perspective about other important parts of your life.

No matter what tomorrow's weight is, take a step back and remember this: On any given day, the number on the scale is exactly what it should be, given what you ate, how much energy you expended in the past few days, the amount of fluid your body is retaining, and other biological influences.

If the scale *has* gone down, be happy, even if you've lost only a small amount of weight. As I tell the dieters I counsel, we celebrate every half-pound loss.

Make Your Graph

Today, you'll create My Weight-Loss Graph (page 174) that'll help you keep weigh-ins in perspective. Even if you weigh yourself as often as daily, keep track of your weight only once a week. On the same day every week, get on the scale and mark down the result in your diet notebook. Over time, you'll fill in a graph that's similar to the one Terri filled out below:

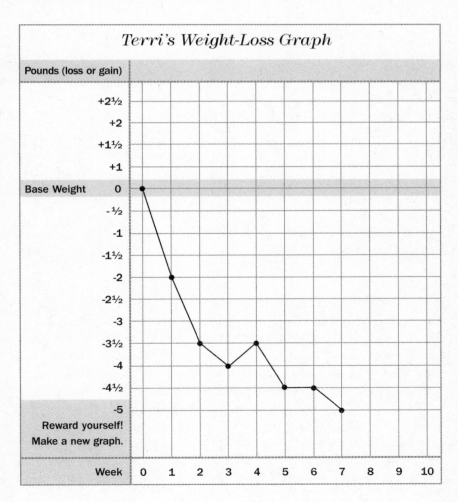

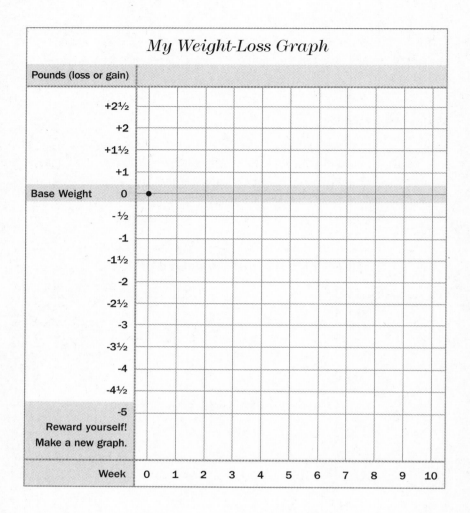

My Weight-Loss Graph

Pounds (loss or gain)	
+2½	
+2	
+1½	
+1	
Base Weight 0	
-½	
-1	
-1½	
-2	
-2½	
-3	
-3½	
-4	
-4½	
-5 Reward yourself! Make a new graph.	
Week 0 1 2 3 4 5 6 7 8 9 10	

Re-create the graph above in your diet notebook, photocopy it, or use a piece of graph paper. When you run out of room on this initial graph (because you've lost more than 5 pounds or dieted for longer than 10 weeks), create a second one, and so on. These graphs will give you an overall sense of your progress. They should help prevent you from focusing too narrowly on the number on the scale on any particular day.

You don't have to write your actual weight on the graph (but you can write it under "Base Weight" if you wish); instead, you'll be tracking how much weight you lose or gain. You'll see that I started off this graph for you, by putting a dot at "0." Tomorrow, you'll note how much your weight has changed and put another dot representing this change on the Week 1 line.

It's important for you to know that virtually no one loses the same amount of weight every single week. Most dieters are like Terri, in that they lose a few pounds fairly quickly and then begin to lose more slowly. *All* dieters have weeks in which their weight either stays the same or increases a little. A typical weight-loss graph resembles a jagged downward slope rather than a straight downward line. Be confident. Overall, your weight *will* go down, but it's unlikely to go down every week.

Your graph can also help you follow your diet program consistently. Many of the dieters I've counseled have told me that they've been motivated to tolerate their cravings partly because they wanted to be able to mark their chart and see the line go down.

Don't expect your weight
*to go down every week—*it won't.

If it turns out that you've gained weight, ask yourself the following questions:

What would I tell a close friend in the same situation? Would I like her less? Would I view her as bad or less worthy or as a failure? Remind yourself that your weight is not a reflection of who you are inside.

What makes me think that I'll lose weight every week? Most people lose some weight, reach a plateau, lose a little more, gain a little back, lose some more, reach another plateau, and so on. Why would I be any different?

What do I need to review with my diet coach? Do I need his or her help in keeping this weight gain in perspective?

what are you thinking?

How do you feel about weighing yourself tomorrow: excited? anxious? fearful? Many dieters tell me that they fear the scale. If you do, too, you might think of excuses for not weighing yourself.

You may need to make Response Cards if you think you may have any of the following thoughts.

Sabotaging Thought: I don't need to weigh myself. I'll know how I'm doing by how my clothes fit.
Helpful Response: It's important to learn the skill of using the number on the scale as information to guide my eating and exercise plans. I'm fooling myself if I think I can regulate myself without this information. If I'm like many dieters, I probably have a tendency to either overestimate or underestimate my weight, both of which can lead to negative consequences.

Sabotaging Thought: I don't want to weigh myself; I think I've gained weight.
Helpful Response: I may or may not have gained weight. If I have, it's not the end of the world, but I do need to know so I can figure out what to do. I need to get over my fear of the scale. It's very important that I not avoid facing facts.

Sabotaging Thought: I'll feel terrible if the number on the scale goes up!
Helpful Response: I'll only feel terrible if I let my sabotaging thoughts convince me that I'm bad or weak for gaining weight. At worst, gaining weight means I might have made mistakes that I can correct during this coming week.

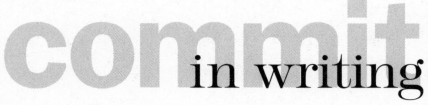
commit in writing

Before I get on the scale tomorrow, I'm going to tell myself: _____

_____

_____

_____

_____ .

> Once I learn to use the number on the
> scale as information, dieting will be easier.

today's to-do list

Check off the tasks you've completed. For any item you haven't completed, record when you're going to complete it.

_____ I read my Advantages, NO CHOICE, It's Not Okay, and Get Back on
Track Response Cards at least twice today.

_____ I read other Response Cards as needed.

_____ I ate slowly, sitting down and noticing every bite.

Circle one: Every time   Most of the time   Some of the time

_____ I gave myself credit for engaging in helpful eating behaviors.

Circle one: Every time   Most of the time   Some of the time

_____ I did spontaneous exercise.

Circle one: Every opportunity   Some of the time   Once or twice   Not at all

_____ I did planned exercise.

_____ I wrote out a food plan for tomorrow.

_____ I monitored everything I ate in writing right after I finished eating.

_____ I ate only to normal fullness.

_____ I made my weight-loss graph.

chapter 8

Week 4

Respond to Sabotaging Thoughts

How are your weight-loss efforts going so far? I hope you're using your Cognitive Therapy skills daily. Some are probably automatic by now. Some are probably still difficult for you. For example, it probably still takes a lot of effort to plan and monitor what you eat, to tolerate cravings, and to use good eating habits. Other skills might still require considerable thought and energy, too. You might need to go back frequently to reread previous material in this book. Stick with it! Your skills will become more and more automatic with each passing day. As you keep practicing, they'll all become second nature. At that point, everything will be much, much easier for you.

This week, you'll continue to build your sense of control and confidence. Each day, you'll identify and respond to the sabotaging thoughts that have previously led you to unplanned eating. You'll learn how to respond to:

Disappointment: *I really wish I could eat this.*
Unfairness: *It's not fair that they can eat that food and I can't.*
Feeling overwhelmed: *This is too hard. I can't keep this up.*

Even though *you now have many new skills to fight sabotaging thoughts and to increase your confidence,* you should expect to face times of doubt and disappointment.

You'll also learn how to identify and respond to sabotaging thoughts, which is one of the most important skills you'll learn in this program. By week's end, you'll be much better equipped to think like a thin person.

day 22

Say, *Oh, Well*, to Disappointment

At some point while you're still losing weight, you'll undoubtedly feel discouraged. It might happen today if the scale doesn't register the number you're hoping to see. It could happen tomorrow or next week when you're with friends and see them eating foods that you can't have. At some point, the disadvantages of dieting will seem to outweigh the advantages. You might feel resentful or even a little rebellious: *Why do I have to do what this book says? There must be an easier way.*

It takes time to change a mindset that took years to form. Even though you now have many new skills to fight sabotaging thoughts and increase your confidence, you should expect to face times of doubt and disappointment.

When this happens, you'll need to remind yourself that you've freely chosen to diet. And having done so, you have another choice as well: You can either make yourself miserable by railing against the fates that "put you in this situation," or you can accept the disadvantages of dieting as a necessary means to an end. Once you truly accept that you need to follow the steps in this program, your struggles will diminish and dieting will become much easier.

Just Say, *Oh, Well*

In 1994, I learned an important lesson about acceptance. That was the year my youngest child was put on an extremely strict diet to control epilepsy. It was a mainstream treatment, called the ketogenic diet, prescribed by his doctor. Thank goodness, it worked! For almost six years (most kids are on it for only two to three years), my son ate three meals a day and no snacks. Each meal consisted mostly of fat—heavy cream and mayonnaise, oil, or butter—with just a small amount of protein and an even smaller amount of carbohydrates. You can imagine why he's my hero. For almost six years, he did not have one bite of candy, cookies, ice cream, or any other treat that contained sugar. He never ate a whole piece of fruit, a whole piece of bread, or more than a couple of chips at a time. He never had seconds or ate between meals. Not once.

You can't stop sabotaging thoughts from arising, but *you* can *respond to them.*

How did we get him to comply with this diet? We used what I call the "Oh, well" technique. Whenever he wanted to eat something he couldn't, he'd get a star on a chart if he just said, *Oh, well*. "Oh, well" means, *I don't like this but I'm going to accept it and move on.*

Within a couple of days, he began to struggle less. Within a week or two, he completely changed his mindset. He knew for certain that there were whole categories of food he couldn't have at all, but he accepted what he had to do and settled down.

The same can happen to you. I don't think it'll happen as quickly, but the more you work toward acceptance, the faster you'll achieve peace of mind about what you have to do. You can't stop your sabotaging thoughts from arising, but you *can* respond to them. When you notice such thoughts as, *It's not fair that I can't eat this,* or *There must be an easier way,* just say to yourself, *Oh, well*. Or in other words, *I don't like this but I'm going to accept it and move on.* Doing so eliminates the struggle, helps you feel better, and allows you to focus your attention elsewhere.

Whenever you find yourself struggling, try saying to yourself, *Oh, well.* These words can also remind you that you've chosen to diet because you want to lose weight. While you may not like dieting, it *is* reality; it *is* what you have to do to reach your goal. Try saying to yourself:

- *I want that doughnut. Oh, well.*
- *I really feel hungry. Oh, well.*
- *I wish I could order a hamburger instead of a salad. Oh, well.*
- *Those chips look so good. Oh, well.*
- *I don't feel like exercising today. Oh, well.*
- *I don't feel like writing down my food plan for tomorrow. Oh, well.*

It's a simple but extremely important concept.

what are you thinking?

Do any of these sabotaging thoughts sound familiar? If so, get ready to make your Response Cards.

Sabotaging Thought: I don't think this will work for me. It seems too simplistic.
Helpful Response: It won't take much time or effort to give this a try. What do I have to lose?

Sabotaging Thought: I don't want to accept the things I have to do. Dieting should be easier.
Helpful Response: I have a choice: I can struggle with what I have to do and feel bad, or I can accept that this is the way it is. It doesn't mean that I like it. There are many things I don't like in my life. I don't particularly like paying bills. I definitely don't like getting up as early as I do for work. I don't like straightening up the house. But I accept them. I don't struggle with these tasks, so they don't cause me much discomfort.

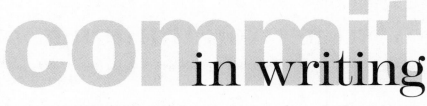

commit in writing

Whenever I find myself struggling, I'm going to: _____
_____
_____
_____
_____
_____
_____ .

Once I accept the changes I have to make,
dieting will be easier.

today's to-do list

It's time for a recap. There are a number of skills you've learned, in addition to the ones that appear in your daily to-do lists. Think about how you're doing with the following:

- Do you need to create more time and energy for dieting?
- Do you need to make any more environmental changes in your kitchen or at work?
- Are you consulting with your diet coach regularly?
- Do you need to skip a meal so you can practice tolerating hunger?
- Do you need to practice leaving food on your plate again?
- Do you need to remind yourself to stop eating before you get overly full?
- If you didn't stick to your food plan, did you get right back on track?

Add anything that you need to work on to this to-do list. Check off the tasks below that you've completed. For any item you haven't completed, record when you're going to complete it.

_____ I read my Advantages, NO CHOICE, It's Not Okay, and Get Back on Track Response Cards at least twice today.

_____ I read other Response Cards as needed.

_____ I ate slowly, sitting down and noticing every bite.

Circle one: Every time   Most of the time   Some of the time

_____ I gave myself credit for engaging in helpful eating behaviors.

Circle one: Every time   Most of the time   Some of the time

_____ I did spontaneous exercise.

Circle one: Every opportunity   Some of the time   Once or twice   Not at all

_____ I did planned exercise.

_____ I wrote out a food plan for tomorrow.

_____ I monitored everything I ate in writing right after I finished eating.

_____ I said, *Oh, well (I don't like this, but I'm going to accept it and move on),* when I wanted something I couldn't have.

_____ I weighed myself, recorded the results on my weight-loss graph, and reported my change in weight to my diet coach.

day 23

Counter the Unfairness Syndrome

Gloria is at work. Her coworkers are eating Girl Scout cookies. She thinks, *It's not fair that I can't eat what everyone else is eating,* and starts to feel resentful. Then she thinks, *I don't care*, and gives in and eats the cookies.

What Gloria doesn't realize is that while it might not seem fair that her coworkers can eat cookies while she can't, it's even less fair that eating the cookies is going to affect her mood and strengthen her giving-in muscle. Even if she doesn't care at the moment, she's going to care very much in a few minutes.

Many dieters give themselves permission to eat when confronted with issues of fairness. You might be one of them. We've all grown up with the idea that life should be fair—but life *isn't* fair. It isn't fair that some people have to struggle with their weight. It isn't fair that some people (due to economic conditions) go hungry every day. It isn't fair that some people die young. Life isn't fair. Dieting isn't fair.

You have a choice when you have thoughts about dieting, eating, food, or weight that start with *It's unfair that....* You can dwell on this negative notion and feel bad, or you can say, *That's true ... It's not fair ... Oh, well.* Then refocus your thoughts on all the advantages in life you have that others don't.

Putting Fairness in Perspective

If the thought that dieting is unfair encourages you to eat, do the following:

Remind yourself why you decided to diet in the first place. Unless you're forced to be on a diet due to a medical reason, you've freely chosen to diet. You don't *have* to diet. You might not feel this way *right at this moment,* but not long ago you strongly felt that the advantages of dieting were worth the hard work. At that time, you felt that the disadvantages of *not* dieting were too severe. Read your Advantages Response Card again.

Make a mental list of the advantages in your life. As compared with many people in the world, you have much more freedom to do what you want, to speak out about what's important to you, to live much of your life as you choose. It's unfair that you have all these freedoms when others don't. Think about other examples of advantages you enjoy.

Create a Response Card. If you constantly think that it's unfair that you have to diet, you need a Response Card to help change your thinking.

This sample card may help you compose your own card:

> Dieting might not be fair, but I have two choices: I can feel sorry for myself, stop following my plan, never reach my goal, and continue to be unhappy with myself. Or I can sympathize with myself but go ahead and do what I know I need to do. Everyone experiences some kind of unfairness in life. This is one of mine. Besides, the greatest unfairness to me would be if I let this excuse prevent me from reaching a goal I strongly want to achieve.

in session
with Dr. Beck

Rosa got so derailed by the notion of unfairness after she'd been dieting for two months that we needed to address this topic in session.

Rosa: So I have to tell you, I had a terrible eating day on Tuesday.

Dr. Beck: Tell me what happened.

Rosa: I was at work, and all the women in my area were eating home-baked cookies. I don't know. It was just so hard. I mean it felt so unfair that they could eat them and I couldn't.

Dr. Beck: So you saw them eating the cookies and you thought, *It's so unfair*. Did you think anything else?

Rosa: Ummm, yeah, that I didn't care, I just really, really wanted to eat some of the cookies.

Dr. Beck: Then what happened?

Rosa: Well, I resisted at first, but one of the women left a bunch of them on a paper plate on the reception desk so people could help themselves, so I took one. And then I took another one. And then I took a third one. And, you know, they were the really fattening kind.

Dr. Beck: And does it still seem unfair that you couldn't eat them?

Rosa: *[sighs]* Well, yeah, a little less so, I guess.

Dr. Beck: And do you still not care that you ate them?

Rosa: No. I feel bad. In fact, I felt bad right away.

Dr. Beck: Rosa, you know you're right that it's unfair that you can't eat them. Do you want to give up on your goal so you can eat them whenever you want?

Rosa: No.

Dr. Beck: Are you sure?

Rosa: Yeah. I really do want to lose weight.

Dr. Beck: I wonder if it would help to think about it like this. It's unfair that you can't eat cookies or, certainly, as many as you'd like. But maybe it would be even more unfair if you ate them and couldn't lose weight. *[pauses]* Which seems more unfair: not eating the cookies or not losing weight?

Rosa: Oh, definitely not losing weight.

Dr. Beck: Okay, so let's make a Response Card. What do you think it should say?

Below is what Rosa wrote on her Response Card:

When it seems unfair to me that I can't eat something, acknowledge that I'm right. Then ask myself, *Which unfairness would I rather have: not being able to eat this or not losing weight?* Then say, "Oh, well," and get on with it.

what are you thinking?

Sabotaging thoughts about the unfairness of dieting may arise sooner or later. Here are some common ones, along with helpful responses.

Sabotaging Thought: It's not fair that I can't eat normally.

Helpful Response: Actually, I probably wasn't eating "normally" before, either. Before I started dieting, I was probably eating too often and too much and choosing too many unhealthy foods. I'm now eating normally for a person who has a goal to lose weight.

Sabotaging Thought: I shouldn't have to deal with this problem.

Helpful Response: I have three choices:

1. I can give up and stay at this weight—or, more likely, continue to gain weight every year.

2. I can diet on and off. Spend some days/months/years eating whatever I want, some days/months/years trying to stick to a diet, and most of the time weighing more than I want to.

3. I can accept the fact that dieting isn't fair and move on, continuing to do what I have to do to lose weight. I'm freely choosing this third option.

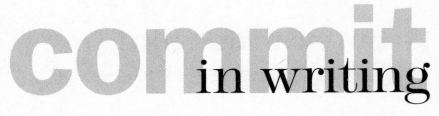

commit in writing

Whenever I hear myself saying that dieting isn't fair, I'm going to: _____

_____

_____

_____

_____.

Once I stop telling myself that dieting
isn't fair, dieting will be easier.

today's to-do list

Check off the tasks you've completed. For any item you haven't completed, record when you're going to complete it.

_____ I read my Advantages, NO CHOICE, It's Not Okay, and Get Back on Track Response Cards at least twice today.

_____ I read other Response Cards as needed.

_____ I ate slowly, sitting down and noticing every bite.

Circle one: Every time   Most of the time   Some of the time

_____ I gave myself credit for engaging in helpful eating behaviors.

Circle one: Every time   Most of the time   Some of the time

_____ I did spontaneous exercise.

Circle one: Every opportunity   Some of the time   Once or twice   Not at all

_____ I did planned exercise.

_____ I wrote out a food plan for tomorrow.

_____ I monitored everything I ate in writing right after I finished eating.

_____ I worked toward accepting what I have to do to lose weight (*Oh, well*).

_____ I created a Response Card to deal with the issue of unfairness.

day 24
Deal with Discouragement

For most people, losing weight starts off easy because their motivation and confidence are high. At some point, though, it begins to get harder. Life intervenes in ways that make sticking to your diet a real effort. Cravings become more intense. And some dieters begin to panic. They have sabotaging thoughts, such as:

- *It shouldn't be this hard.*
- *I'll never be able to keep this up.*
- *I don't want to do this anymore.*

It's normal to feel overwhelmed or discouraged at times. It's natural to have doubts about whether you can keep doing what you know you have to do, but it's not okay to let these thoughts overwhelm you. When you have discouraging thoughts, you have a choice. You can allow them to erode your motivation, give up, and abandon your goal. Or you can vigorously respond to these sabotaging thoughts, feel better, become more motivated, and continue to work toward your goal.

It's important to remind yourself that you *can* do what you need to do! Remember, dieting *does* get easier. Today's task will help you persevere with your efforts even when the going gets tough.

Finding Encouragement

To motivate yourself, especially in the face of self-doubt, do the following:

Read your Advantages Response Card more often. It'll probably help to rewrite this card, thinking about each item carefully. Add any new advantages that you hadn't written previously.

Add up the difficult hours. Many dieters I've counseled have wanted to give up at one point or another. They've come to me and said, "I had *such* a hard week. I don't know if I want to do this any more." Then they'd tell me about some struggle they went through to stay on their diet.

It's interesting how the memory of these struggles tainted their whole week. As it turned out, most of them struggled for between 20 minutes and a couple of hours once or twice during the week. For the other 164 hours of the week, they *hadn't* struggled. During most of these other hours, they hadn't even *thought* about dieting. Yet they all initially reported that the entire *week* had been intolerable.

Remind yourself that dieting is not difficult
most of the hours of the week.

Figure out how many minutes or hours you actually struggled in the past week versus how many hours you actually felt neutral or positive. Think about how much time you weren't even *thinking* about food or dieting.

Focus on what you can do today. Thinking too far into the future is incredibly unhelpful. Every time you find yourself thinking, *I can't keep this up for a month, a year, or longer,* tell yourself, *Forget the long term ... Focus on today ... I know I can continue to do what I need to do today ... If it's hard tomorrow, I'll deal with it then.* Make a Response Card to remind yourself of all this.

what are you thinking?

When you feel overwhelmed about the future, you may notice some of the following sabotaging thoughts. Prepare for them now by creating Response Cards.

Sabotaging Thought: I feel overwhelmed. This program is way too involved. I can't do it!

Helpful Response: This book will help me, step-by-step. I don't have to learn everything in one day. I can reread and practice. I can ask my diet coach to help me.

Sabotaging Thought: These tasks are too hard. I don't want to keep on doing these things.

Helpful Response: I'm just feeling overwhelmed at the moment. It doesn't always seem this hard. Later on today or tomorrow, it'll probably feel easier again.

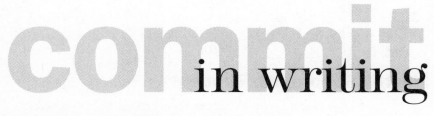

commit in writing

Whenever I feel overwhelmed or discouraged, I'm going to: _____

_____

_____

_____

_____ .

Once I focus only on what I have
to do today, dieting will be easier.

today's to-do list

Check off the tasks you've completed. For any item you haven't completed, record when you're going to complete it.

_____ I read my Advantages, NO CHOICE, It's Not Okay, and Get Back on Track Response Cards at least twice today.

_____ I read other Response Cards as needed.

_____ I ate slowly, sitting down and noticing every bite.

Circle one: Every time   Most of the time   Some of the time

_____ I gave myself credit for engaging in helpful eating behaviors.

Circle one: Every time   Most of the time   Some of the time

_____ I did spontaneous exercise.

Circle one: Every opportunity   Some of the time   Once or twice   Not at all

_____ I did planned exercise.

_____ I wrote out a food plan for tomorrow.

_____ I monitored everything I ate in writing right after I finished eating.

_____ I worked toward accepting what I have to do to lose weight (*Oh, well*).

_____ I prepared for feeling overwhelmed and discouraged.

day 25

Identify Sabotaging Thoughts

You've been reading a lot about sabotaging thoughts in this book. I've included the most common ones that I've heard from dieters over the years. I've also found, though, that every dieter has additional sabotaging thoughts. It's important for you to learn to recognize your unique sabotaging thoughts and to respond to them effectively.

As I've mentioned before, eating doesn't happen automatically. Before you take that first bite of something you didn't plan to eat, you almost always have a thought or a series of thoughts. Once you identify and respond to those thoughts, you'll be better able to control your eating.

Think About It

Carry your diet notebook and a pen (or your PDA) with you for a few days. Mark down your sabotaging thoughts as you identify them. You might not always notice these thoughts right away because your attention might be focused on how you're feeling. If you notice that you're tempted to eat something that you're not supposed to eat, ask yourself, *What was just going through my mind?* or *What was I just thinking?*

Sometimes, you'll be able to identify your thoughts easily. Other times, you won't. If you're not sure what you were thinking, see "Common Diet-Related Sabotaging Thoughts" on the facing page. If this list doesn't jog your memory, try to figure out what you definitely were *not* thinking. For example, if you have an urge to eat something you hadn't planned to eat, ask yourself if you were thinking about any of the following:

- How unappetizing the food looks and smells?
- How glad you are that you're not supposed to eat it?
- How easy it'll be to resist it?

You'll undoubtedly answer in the negative, followed by your actual thought: *I was thinking I really want to eat it!*

Write each thought you identify in your diet notebook. For now, don't worry about what to do about these thoughts. You'll learn how to respond to them in a couple of days.

common diet-related sabotaging thoughts

To help you identify your sabotaging thoughts, here are examples of common thoughts among the dieters I've counseled:

Dieting is too hard.

I don't care.

It's okay to eat this.

I'm being punished.

It's not fair.

I'm not going to let anyone tell me what I can and can't eat.

I deserve to eat this.

I'll just eat these crumbs.

I should be able to do what I want.

I can't resist.

I really want it.

I'm really hungry.

I have no willpower.

It's not that fattening.

I'll make up for it later.

It'll go to waste if I don't eat it.

I should eat it because it's free.

Everyone else is eating.

I don't want to disappoint or inconvenience [fill in the blank].

I'm stressed/tired/sad/bored/upset.

It's a special occasion.

I'm treating myself.

I can start dieting again tomorrow.

I'll never lose weight anyway.

No one will know.

I'll end up eating it eventually.

what are you thinking?

If you're concerned about your ability to learn this skill, read the sabotaging thoughts and responses below.

Sabotaging Thought: I don't know if I can figure out what I'm thinking.

Helpful Response: It's not that crucial to figure it out right now. It's a skill I'll get better at over time. Meanwhile, I can reread relevant parts of the book to jog my memory whenever I need to.

Sabotaging Thought: I'm not thinking anything when I stray from my diet. It just happens.

Helpful Response: Eating is not automatic. I just try to ignore my thoughts so I can eat. The next time I'm tempted to stray, I'm going to look for some sabotaging thought that gives me permission, such as, *It's okay to eat this because....*

commit in writing

Whenever I have a desire to go off my diet, I'm going to: _____
_____
_____.

(I hope you wrote, "stop and look for sabotaging thoughts.")

Once I get good at identifying my sabotaging thoughts (so I can respond to them), dieting will be easier.

today's to-do list

Check off the tasks you've completed. For any item you haven't completed, record when you're going to complete it.

_____ I read my Advantages, NO CHOICE, It's Not Okay, and Get Back on Track Response Cards at least twice today.

_____ I read other Response Cards as needed.

_____ I ate slowly, sitting down and noticing every bite.

Circle one: Every time   Most of the time   Some of the time

_____ I gave myself credit for engaging in helpful eating behaviors.

Circle one: Every time   Most of the time   Some of the time

_____ I did spontaneous exercise.

Circle one: Every opportunity   Some of the time   Once or twice   Not at all

_____ I did planned exercise.

_____ I wrote out a food plan for tomorrow.

_____ I monitored everything I ate in writing right after I finished eating.

_____ I worked toward accepting what I have to do to lose weight (*Oh, well*).

_____ I identified and wrote down one or more sabotaging thoughts.

day 26
Recognize Thinking Mistakes

I t's important to realize that thoughts are just ideas, not necessarily truths. Your thoughts about anything might be completely true, partially true, or completely false. For example, if you haven't eaten all day and pass by people who are eating pizza, you might think, *That looks so good ... I'm so hungry,* which might well be true. In fact, this thought isn't necessarily a problem. The problematic one comes next. The thought, *I have to have some,* is *not* true. But if you're like most people, you probably accept this last thought as true, without really thinking about it—at least at that moment.

Common Thinking Errors

There are nine common thinking mistakes people make when dieting:

Thinking Mistake #1: All or Nothing Thinking
You see things in only two categories when there's really a middle ground.
Examples:
- *Either I'm completely on my diet or I'm off my diet.*
- *Either I'm 100 percent successful or I'm a failure and may as well give up dieting.*

Thinking Mistake #2: Negative Fortune Telling
You predict the future negatively, without considering other possible outcomes.
Examples:
- *Since I didn't lose weight this week, I'll never be able to lose weight.*
- *Since I gave into that craving, I'll never be able to tolerate cravings.*

Thinking Mistake #3: Overly Positive Fortune Telling
You predict the future too positively, without considering other possible outcomes.
Examples:
- *I'll be able to eat just a little bit of this food I crave, feel satisfied, and stop.*
- *It's okay if I just estimate the amount of food I'm supposed to have instead of measuring it. I'll still lose weight.*

Thinking Mistake #4: Emotional Reasoning

You think your ideas must be true even though objective evidence says not.

Examples:

- *Since I feel like a failure for having strayed, I really must be a failure.*
- *I feel like I just have to have something sweet right now.*

Thinking Mistake #5: Mind Reading

You're sure of what others are thinking, even in the absence of compelling data.

Examples:

- *People will think I'm strange if I don't drink alcohol at the party.*
- *She'll think I'm rude if I don't try the brownies she baked.*

Thinking Mistake #6: Self-Deluding Thinking

You rationalize by telling yourself things you don't really believe at other times.

Examples:

- *If no one sees me eating, it doesn't count.*
- *It won't matter if I give in to my cravings.*

Thinking Mistake #7: Unhelpful Rules

You mandate actions without taking circumstances into consideration.

Examples:

- *I can't waste food.*
- *I can't inconvenience my family by cooking healthier meals or getting the junk food out of the house.*

Thinking Mistake #8: Justification

You link two unrelated concepts (to justify your eating).

Examples:

- *I deserve to eat this because I'm so stressed out.*
- *It's okay to eat this because it's free.*

Thinking Mistake #9: Exaggerated Thinking

You make a situation seem greater or worse than it really is.

Examples:

- *I can't stand this craving.*
- *I have no willpower.*

Pull out your diet notebook and turn to the sabotaging thoughts you identified yesterday. Write down the thinking mistake that corresponds to each thought. (Some thoughts might contain more than one thinking error.)

what are you thinking?

Try not to get self-critical as you identify your errors in thinking. If you do become critical of yourself, create a Response Card.

Sabotaging Thought: I must be stupid for making thinking mistakes.

Helpful Response: There's nothing wrong with me. Everyone has distorted thinking from time to time. It has nothing to do with intelligence. It just means I'm human. The important thing is to learn what to do about my thinking mistakes. I'm taking the first step right now by identifying them.

commit in writing

When I notice sabotaging thoughts, I'll: _____
_____
_____.

(I hope you wrote, "identify the thinking mistakes that go with them.")

Once I can readily see the mistakes in my thinking, dieting will be easier.

today's to-do list

Check off the tasks you've completed. For any item you haven't completed, record when you're going to complete it.

_____ I read my Advantages, NO CHOICE, It's Not Okay, and Get Back on Track Response Cards at least twice today.

_____ I read other Response Cards as needed.

_____ I ate slowly, sitting down and noticing every bite.

   Circle one: Every time   Most of the time   Some of the time

_____ I gave myself credit for engaging in helpful eating behaviors.

   Circle one: Every time   Most of the time   Some of the time

_____ I did spontaneous exercise.

   Circle one: Every opportunity   Some of the time   Once or twice   Not at all

_____ I did planned exercise.

_____ I wrote out a food plan for tomorrow.

_____ I monitored everything I ate in writing right after I finished eating.

_____ I worked toward accepting what I have to do to lose weight (*Oh, well*).

_____ I identified the thinking mistakes that correspond to my common sabotaging thoughts.

day 27

Master the Seven Question Technique

You now have your list of sabotaging thoughts and thinking mistakes. Today, you'll create additional Response Cards to help you more effectively reply to these thoughts. You'll read these cards at a set time every day, ideally when you read your Advantages Response Card. You'll also pull them out whenever you need them. Over time, as you practice these ideas again and again, you'll begin to automatically respond to your sabotaging thoughts, even without the cards.

How to Make Your Cards

As you look through your notebook and examine your common sabotaging thoughts, reflect on each one by asking yourself, *What do I wish I could remember the next time I have this thought?* Write down your response using the technique below. Not all questions will apply to every sabotaging thought, but write down responses to the ones that do.

The Seven Question Technique

1. What kind of thinking error could I be making? (Review Day 26 on pages 195–198 to help you figure out the answer to this question.)
2. What evidence is there that this thought might not be true (or not completely true)?
3. Is there an alternative explanation or another way of viewing this?
4. What is the most realistic outcome of this situation?
5. What is the effect of my believing this thought and what could be the effect of changing my thinking?
6. What would I tell [a close friend or family member] if he/she were in this situation and had this thought?
7. What should I do now?

Over time, as you practice these ideas
again and again, *you'll begin to automatically
respond to your sabotaging thoughts,*
even without Response Cards.

Here is an example of how Eric used the Seven Question Technique to design a card for himself. He frequently had the thought, *I can't control myself,* when he was eating out and friends offered him dessert.

Sabotaging thought: I can't control my eating.

1. What kind of thinking error could I be making?
Exaggeration.

2. What's the evidence that this thought might not be true?
I control myself all the time in other areas, especially at work. I do lots of things I don't want to do and don't do lots of things I do want to do. In fact, I control myself a lot when it comes to dieting.

3. What's an alternative explanation or another way of viewing this?
That I can control myself, but I don't want to right now.

4. What's the most realistic outcome?
I'll stop craving once I firmly tell myself, NO CHOICE, and get busy with something else.

5. What's the effect of believing this thought and what could be the effect of changing my thinking?
If I believe it, I'll give in to this craving, feel terrible afterwards, maybe not lose weight this week, and be at greater risk the next time I have a craving. If I change my thinking, I won't give in and I'll lose weight!

6. What would I tell my friend Marissa if she were in this situation and had this thought?
I'd tell her that she could decide to control herself if she wanted to and that I don't want her to feel bad later.

7. What should I do?
Tell myself, NO CHOICE. Turn my attention away from the food. Focus on the conversation. If needed, go to the restroom and read my Response Cards!

Based on his answers, Eric created the following Response Card:

It's not that I can't control myself. It's that I don't want to control myself right at this moment. This craving is strong, but there are a lot of things I can do to counteract it. I'll be glad if I do.

There will be times when you'll need to use the Seven Question Technique to write your Response Cards. At other times, it might be helpful just to read short, direct statements, such as the following examples:

- I'd rather be thin.
- Get out of the kitchen—now!
- No excuses!
- This is just a craving! It'll go away! Don't eat!

Short commands like these are also good to repeat to yourself (silently if you're around other people) at the first sign of craving.

Try writing one or more Response Cards of your own now, using the Seven Question Technique. Read these new cards along with your other cards at least once or twice a day. As you identify additional sabotaging thoughts, create more Response Cards.

what are you thinking?

Some of the dieters I counsel resist making their cards at first because of such sabotaging thoughts as, *I can't do this ... I don't know what to write.* Like any skill, creating cards based on the Seven Question Technique becomes easier over time. If you get stuck, ask your diet coach for help. Also, review the dozens of helpful responses that appear throughout this book.

If you continue to feel resistant about creating Response Cards, be sure to apply the Seven Question Technique to the sabotaging thoughts that are getting in your way.

So what are you thinking? Perhaps one of the following sabotaging thoughts sounds familiar right about now.

Sabotaging Thought: This is a lot of work. It might not even help.
Helpful Response: That might be true, but I might as well do everything I can to lose weight. When I'm thinner, I'll be so glad I put in the hard work today.

Sabotaging Thought: I've always thought this way. I don't think I can change my thinking.
Helpful Response: This is a skill that I can learn. It wasn't easy learning how to drive a car or to ride a bike, but I eventually got good at those things. If I practice, I can get good at responding to my sabotaging thinking.

commit in writing

I'll look at the sabotaging thoughts I've identified so far and:_____

_____

_____

_____.

(I hope you wrote, "create Response Cards to read daily.")

Once I accept the fact that I have to monitor my eating in this way, dieting will be easier.

today's to-do list

Check off the tasks you've completed. For any item you haven't completed, record when you're going to complete it.

_____ I read my Advantages, NO CHOICE, It's Not Okay, and Get Back on Track Response Cards at least twice today.

_____ I read other Response Cards as needed.

_____ I ate slowly, sitting down and noticing every bite.

Circle one: Every time   Most of the time   Some of the time

_____ I gave myself credit for engaging in helpful eating behaviors.

Circle one: Every time   Most of the time   Some of the time

_____ I did spontaneous exercise.

Circle one: Every opportunity   Some of the time   Once or twice   Not at all

_____ I did planned exercise.

_____ I wrote out a food plan for tomorrow.

_____ I monitored everything I ate in writing right after I finished eating.

_____ I worked toward accepting what I have to do to lose weight (*Oh, well*).

_____ I used the Seven Question Technique to make Response Cards.

day 28

Get Ready to Weigh In

Tomorrow marks the end of your second week of dieting. When you get up in the morning, step on the scale. Wear the same weight clothing as you wore last week. Calculate your change in weight, add a new dot on your weight-loss graph (page 174), and connect the dots.

Don't even think about trying to skimp on food today in order to have a more favorable outcome tomorrow. You need to squarely face whatever number you see on the scale. And eating too little today might set you up for going overboard in the following day or two.

what are you thinking?

Sabotaging thoughts about weighing yourself might surface tomorrow if you're disappointed by the number you see on the scale. Prepare yourself today for these thoughts by making Response Cards.

Based on the experiences of the dieters I've counseled, I can guess that your thoughts might go in one of three directions, depending on the number that appears on the scale.

Scenario No. 1: You lost what you consider to be a lot of weight.
Sabotaging Thought: That's great! I'm going to keep losing weight fast!
Helpful Response: Yes, it's great that I've lost this much weight. I did a good job following my diet this week. But I probably won't continue to lose weight this quickly.

Scenario No. 2: You lost what you think is too little weight.
Sabotaging Thought: I've worked so hard, and the weight I've lost is just a drop in the bucket.
Helpful Response: My weight is going down. That's good! It means that what I've been doing is working. I should celebrate each half-pound weight loss.

Scenario No. 3: You don't lose weight, or you gain weight.
Sabotaging Thought: I can't believe this! See, I just can't lose weight.
Helpful Response: My weight might be up temporarily for hormonal or other reasons. If my weight doesn't go down next week, I'll call my coach and see if she can meet me to go over my food plans. Maybe I made some mistakes. Maybe I need to decrease my caloric intake or exercise more. I just need to stay problem solving–oriented.

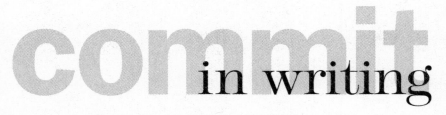
commit in writing

Before I step on the scale tomorrow, I'm going to remind myself: _____

_____

_____

_____.

Once I learn to use the scale
as information to guide my efforts,
dieting will be easier.

today's to-do list

Check off the tasks you've completed. For any item you haven't completed, record when you're going to complete it.

_____ I read my Advantages, NO CHOICE, It's Not Okay, and Get Back on Track Response Cards at least twice today.

_____ I read other Response Cards as needed.

_____ I ate slowly, sitting down and noticing every bite.

Circle one: Every time   Most of the time   Some of the time

_____ I gave myself credit for engaging in helpful eating behaviors.

Circle one: Every time   Most of the time   Some of the time

_____ I did spontaneous exercise.

Circle one: Every opportunity   Some of the time   Once or twice   Not at all

_____ I did planned exercise.

_____ I wrote out a food plan for tomorrow.

_____ I monitored everything I ate in writing right after I finished eating.

_____ I worked toward accepting what I have to do to lose weight (*Oh, well*).

_____ I prepared for my weigh-in tomorrow.

chapter 9

Week 5

Overcome Challenges

By now, you should be experiencing some of the wonderful benefits of this program. Have you figured out that hunger is never an emergency? That you can withstand cravings? That you can tolerate the discomfort of not eating when you're not supposed to?

These are all very important things you've learned. I expect that many of the new habits you're developing—such as monitoring what you're eating—don't feel as time-consuming now as they did when you started. Equally important, you're probably much better at noticing sabotaging thoughts almost as soon as they arise and can respond to some almost instantly. You've begun to master some essential Cognitive Therapy techniques.

Now, it's time to move forward and learn how to prepare for both expected and unexpected challenges. Have you ever stopped dieting because you were on vacation? Have you ever "blown it" at a restaurant or party? Have you ever eaten in response to social pressure, only to feel bad about it later? How often do you eat for emotional reasons because you're upset or bored? This week, you'll learn how to stay in control during challenging situations. What you learn this week will allow you to diet and enjoy the pleasures of life.

*How often **do you eat for emotional reasons** because you're upset or bored?*

day 29

Resist Food Pushers

M any of the dieters I've counseled have told me they "had to eat" to avoid hurting someone's feelings, even though they knew it meant straying from their diet. Bill, for example, told me that he felt he had to eat whatever his wife prepared for dinner. Allison told me she always ate a piece of whatever baked goods her coworkers brought to work. Melissa never refused the desserts her mother-in-law made. They all were certain that even a polite refusal of food would offend the other person.

Do you find you have a similar problem? If so, you probably have two notions that get in the way: The first is that other people's desire to have you eat their food is more important than your desire to lose weight. The second is that it's wrong to stick up for yourself (at least where food is concerned), especially if it means disappointing someone else. I'd like you to think about these two ideas in a different way:

- You're entitled to work toward your goal of losing weight as long as you're not maliciously trying to make someone feel bad.

- It's okay to disappoint others. Disappointment is a normal part of life. Their disappointment most likely will be mild and fleeting.

In order to make a point about social eating, I often tell dieters about an experience I recently had. They usually have interesting reactions to the story. I wonder what yours will be. Here's what happened:

While I was writing this book, I attended a dessert reception given in my honor, following a workshop I had presented in another city. My gracious hostess had obviously spent a lot of time and effort preparing for the reception: buying food, baking lots of desserts, and beautifully laying it all out on a buffet table. I ate only a few small pieces of sliced fruit, despite her gentle urging, "Wouldn't you like to try this? Are you sure you've had enough?" Each time she urged me to eat, I replied, "Thank you. It all looks so delicious, but I'm fine with just this fruit."

Did this make my hostess feel bad? Should I have eaten more, since she'd worked so hard to make the food? Was it rude of me to eat so little?

Some dieters I've told this story to thought I'd done exactly the right thing. A few of them, though, were rather taken aback. They were sure that I'd either insulted my hostess or made her feel major disappointment.

I actually got to check out my hostess's reaction when I saw her about a month later at a national conference. I explained that I'd told the people I was working with about the reception. I asked her what she'd thought when I declined her wonderful desserts. She looked a little puzzled and, as I'd suspected, said that she didn't remember that I hadn't eaten very much.

Then we talked about the subject of social-eating pressure. She told me that for years she'd felt obliged to overeat whenever she visited her aunt in India. Finally, a couple of years ago, she called her aunt in advance and told her that she was looking forward to visiting her but that she wouldn't be able to eat much because she was watching her diet. Her aunt said fine, she didn't mind at all; she'd just be happy to see her niece.

What is the message in these stories? We often feel that we're hurting people's feelings when we refuse their offer of food when, in fact, they either feel neutral or, at worst, have a mild reaction. If you find that you're assuming others will be disappointed if you turn down food, ask yourself:

- *Won't I be disappointed if I accept the food and stray from my food plan?*
- *Why is it more important for me to please them than it is to do what is best for me?*

Or think about it another way. If you were a vegetarian, would you eat meat just to please someone? If you were on a special diet for medical reasons, would you abandon that diet just to spare someone's feelings? You're entitled to do what is right for you, as long as you're polite (but firm, if necessary). People who give you a hard time are the ones who are being unreasonable, not you.

in session with Dr. Beck

Two days after the dessert reception, I told the story to Julie, a dieter with whom I was working. Her first reaction was that I had been inconsiderate.

Julie: Wasn't your hostess offended? Weren't you being rude?

Dr. Beck: I don't think she was offended. She didn't look upset. It's possible she was a little disappointed.

Julie: But isn't that terrible?

Dr. Beck: To disappoint her? No. I was polite. I didn't *intentionally* try to make her feel bad.

Julie: But she'd gone to so much trouble!

Dr. Beck: That's true. But if I'd eaten the desserts, I'd have gone beyond what I was comfortable eating. I had just come from dinner. I wasn't particularly hungry, and I'd already eaten more than I usually eat.

Julie: But you might have made her feel bad.

Dr. Beck: That's possible. Let's assume you're right. Let's assume she was disappointed. How major a disappointment do you think it was in the big scheme of things?

Julie: [thinks] Not that much, I guess.

Dr. Beck: And how long do you think she stayed disappointed? There was a large room full of guests, and most of them were busy eating.

Julie: [sighs] I guess she probably didn't think about it that much.

Dr. Beck: I think you're right. Even if she were disappointed, I think it was very mild and didn't last for long. You see, I did this quick mental calculation: If I ate the desserts, what would be the benefit to her versus the cost to me? I decided the benefit to her would be very small and the benefit to me of *not* eating would be much greater. This is pretty much how I calculate it no matter who is offering me food.

Julie: So you're saying it really is okay to turn down people?

Dr. Beck: About food? Absolutely.

How to Say No

Prepare now to turn down someone the next time you're offered something to eat. Here's how:

Create a sense of entitlement about turning down requests to eat. Look at My Cost Analysis of Eating Chart on page 211. To fill it in, think of a specific situation where someone might offer you food. What are the costs to you of accepting the offer? It could make you:

- Go off your scheduled meal plan.
- Eat more than you really want.
- Feel subservient to others.
- Feel out of control.
- Stop losing or even gain weight.
- Overeat or develop a craving.
- Feel bad about yourself.

Before you write down the costs to someone else, think about how you would react if people turned down food that you'd offered, particularly if you knew they were trying to lose weight. How bad would you feel? How long would that negative feeling last? I wonder if any reasonable person would have more than a temporary, mildly negative reaction.

Prepare your initial response. What will you say the next time someone offers you food? Write what you plan to say in your notebook or on a Response Card. For many people, "No, thanks," or "No, thank you, it looks delicious, but I'm fine," will probably suffice. You don't have to explain that you're on a diet or watching what you're eating if you don't want to. If it's appropriate and if you want, you can always say, "Thank you, it looks really good. Could I take a little piece home for later?"

Visualize your plan in action. Who will most likely push food on you in the near future? Where will you be? Who else will be around? What foods will be involved? Try to imagine the scene. See him or her offering you the food. Hear yourself saying, "No, thank you." Think about what this person might say next and how you might respond. See the person turn away and offer the food to someone else. Visualize giving yourself lots of credit and feeling proud of yourself for being politely assertive about your needs.

If you haven't had much practice in turning down food, you might get a little nervous the first time you try it. It'll definitely get easier to do over time, as you see that nothing terrible happens.

special advice to persistent food pushers

Most people will accept a simple, "No, thank you," and stop asking you to eat. But some people, as you may already know, will not.

To prepare your response to persistent food pushers, think of a good role model, someone you know who is nicely assertive about his or her needs. (If no one comes to mind, think of a celebrity you know about.) What would he or she say if in your situation? The dialogue would probably go something like this:

Persistent food pusher: Have a piece of birthday cake.

Role model: Thank you, but no.

Persistent food pusher: But it's my birthday! You *have* to have a piece!

Role model: I know, and the cake looks so good, but I really have to say no.

Persistent food pusher: Oh, come on. A little taste won't hurt.

Role model: No, really no, thank you anyway.

Persistent food pusher: You're hurting my feelings.

Role model: I'm not turning down the cake to make you feel bad. I just don't want any right now.

My Cost Analysis of Eating Chart

Costs to Me of Eating	Costs to Other Person of My Not Eating

what are you thinking?

What's your reaction to my story? If you're like Julie (pages 208–209), perhaps some of these sabotaging thoughts entered your mind. If so, pay close attention to the responses.

Sabotaging Thought: If I don't eat, _____ will be upset or insulted.
Helpful Response: I wouldn't be upset if someone else didn't want to eat. If others don't like it, that's their problem, not mine. I don't have to please them or justify myself. I don't want to let their reaction (or my prediction about their reaction) get in my way.

_____

Sabotaging Thought: I have to please others by eating, no matter what the cost is to me.
Helpful Response: I have to work toward my goal, especially since the cost to others is momentary and minor. My not eating won't spoil their entire year. It's good for me to say no.

commit in writing

When someone tries to push food on me, I'll: _____
_____
_____
_____.

Once I firmly believe I'm
entitled to say no to food pushers,
dieting will be easier.

today's to-do list

By now, many of the program tasks should feel automatic. Before you complete today's to-do list, however, think about whether you're still regularly:

- Creating enough time and energy for dieting
- Consulting with your diet coach
- Reminding yourself that hunger is never an emergency
- Using anti-craving techniques
- Eating only to normal fullness

If you're not, add these tasks to today's to-do list. Check off the tasks you've completed. For any item you haven't completed, record when you're going to complete it.

_____ I read my Advantages, NO CHOICE, It's Not Okay, and Get Back on Track Response Cards at least twice today.

_____ I read other Response Cards as needed.

_____ I ate slowly, sitting down and noticing every bite.

Circle one: Every time   Most of the time   Some of the time

_____ I gave myself credit for engaging in helpful eating behaviors.

Circle one: Every time   Most of the time   Some of the time

_____ I wrote a food plan for tomorrow and monitored everything I ate in writing right after I finished eating.

_____ I did spontaneous and planned exercise.

_____ I dealt effectively with issues of unfairness and discouragement.

_____ I decided how I'll respond to food pushers.

_____ I weighed myself, recorded the results on my weight-loss graph, and reported my change in weight to my diet coach.

day 30

Stay in Control When Eating Out

When you go to a restaurant, family gathering, holiday celebration, or other special event, you'll encounter lots of triggers: the sight and smell of food, people eating and drinking, people offering you food and drink, a festive atmosphere. Many people apply special eating and drinking rules to special occasions. They give themselves permission to indulge.

That's why so many dieters come undone.

Plan to Eat Out

Today, you'll create a plan for eating out and set a date to implement this plan at a restaurant some time this week. Sticking to your diet every time you eat out or while celebrating is a skill that requires preparation and practice. Here's what you should do to get ready:

- **Choose a suitable day and place.** Pick a day this week when you're not particularly stressed and plan to eat at a slightly earlier time than usual, so you won't be too hungry. Select a restaurant that serves foods permitted on your plan.
- **Go with a friend.** Choose someone whom you know won't try to push food on you. Perhaps you should go with your diet coach.
- **Plan in advance how much you're going to eat.** It's fine to eat a little more than usual—perhaps up to 25 percent more calories than you ordinarily would have eaten for that meal. If you don't eat out very often, the extra food shouldn't appreciably slow down your rate of weight loss.
- **Plan what you're going to eat.** Check to see if the restaurant has a menu posted on a Web site. Think about which foods you might eat and the size of portions you should consume.
- **Anticipate the sabotaging thoughts you might have.** You might think, for example, *It's okay to eat more than I've planned because ... everyone else is eating a lot/ I rarely get to eat these foods/it won't hurt/I can start again tomorrow/I should eat more to get my money's worth.* Make Response Cards to read before you go and bring them with you in case you need them. Make sure to review and bring along your Advantages Response Card, too.
- **Plan how you'll tolerate cravings.** What can you say to yourself? What can you do? Review Day 13 to remind yourself of the mindset and behavioral techniques you can use (pages 127–134). For example, if you start craving, you might need to distance yourself from the food by taking a short walk through the restaurant, by going outside, or by going to the restroom to read your Response Cards.

- **When your food arrives, portion off the food you can eat.** Immediately push the extra food not on your food plan to one side of your plate. Or put it on your bread plate, if you prefer.

- **Assess your success.** Once you get back home, think about how you did. If you weren't able to follow your food plan, what will you do differently next time? Beware of self-critical thoughts. If you had trouble, the task was just too challenging. Try it again and prepare yourself better before you go.

- **If you did well but feel disgruntled because you couldn't eat everything you wanted, work on your sabotaging thoughts.** Give yourself great credit for following through with your food plan and work on acceptance: *Oh, well, I couldn't eat the way I used to eat. But I do really want to lose weight so it's good that I limited myself.*

tip!
If you dine out without overeating, give yourself lots of credit. But don't undo your good eating when you get home. Some dieters tell themselves, *I was so good ... Now I deserve to treat myself,* and then eat an unplanned snack. Of course, it's fine to plan in advance to eat something when you get home. I purposely avoid eating dessert when I'm out because I look forward to my evening snack every night. If I've already eaten dessert, I won't be able to have that snack.

The more you practice eating out, the easier it'll be. If not this time, eventually you'll leave a restaurant or event and say to yourself, *I'm so glad I didn't overeat.* When I told this to dieters I've worked with, most didn't believe me at first, saying "I can't *imagine* that happening. I think I'll *always* feel deprived." But they do get to this point. They feel good for remaining in control.

Dining-Out Strategies

The following strategies can help you to stay in control while eating out. As you read them, watch out for sabotaging thoughts, such as, *I couldn't do that.* The dieters I've counseled and I routinely do these things—and we feel glad that we do.

Tell the waiter how you'd like your food prepared. Don't hesitate to ask for substitutions or other special arrangements. Many diners routinely make such requests, and waiters are accustomed to accommodating them. The worst thing that could happen is that they can't do what you've requested, but in my experience that doesn't occur very often. Watch out for sabotaging thoughts such as, *I'm creating too much trouble for them.* Read "What Are You Thinking?" on page 218 to prepare for these thoughts ahead of time.

Sticking to your diet every time
you eat out or while celebrating is a skill that
requires preparation and practice.

Order smaller portions. Order an appetizer as an entrée or ask if you can get an appetizer portion of an entrée. Watch out for sabotaging thoughts, such as, *My dining companions will be critical of me if I eat so little.*

If you're eating at a buffet or family-style restaurant, look at all food options before filling your plate. Of the foods allowed on your diet plan, which look the most appealing? Would you feel more satisfied with very small tastes of several different foods or with larger portions of just a few foods? Make a decision and then put food on your plate. Remind yourself that this is it—no seconds. If you feel disappointed, say, *Oh, well, I'd rather be able to eat more, but I'm moving on … I'd rather lose weight even more.*

Practice what you know. Eat slowly and notice every bite, even if you're distracted by your companions and the environment.

When you're finished eating, make it final. Arrange the flatware so that the handles rest in the remaining food. If you can, put your paper napkin on your plate. Push away your plate.

Change Your Mindset About Parties, Celebrations, and Special Events

If you want to lose weight and maintain it for your lifetime, you need to develop a different attitude toward celebrating than you've had before. If you're like most people, you have an idea that is quite strong in your mind: *I'm entitled to make exceptions for special circumstances.* There are three difficulties associated with this notion:

1. You're likely to encounter special circumstances repeatedly. Think about all the special circumstances that could arise just in the next year: meals at the home of friends and family, parties, holiday celebrations, luncheons, showers, weddings, retirement parties, office parties, business-related events, charity events, religious occasions, receptions, benefits—the list could go on and on. If you give yourself permission to make exceptions, you could easily overeat at all of them.

2. You might go overboard in making exceptions. Instead of just eating a small to moderate amount more at a special meal (perhaps a couple of hundred more calories), you could easily eat *much* more. For example, if your

special advice for business dinners

usual dinner is 600 calories, you could end up eating 200 percent more—or a total of 1,800 calories. Once you go over your planned limit, you may think, *I've already blown it ... I may as well eat whatever I want.*

3. You might find it difficult to return to restricted eating once the event is over. You might have sabotaging thoughts, such as, *It was really fun to eat whatever I wanted ... I really liked not restricting myself.* You might lose sight of why it has been so important to you to lose weight—and you might stop following the steps in this program. Or you might have such sabotaging thoughts as, *I really lost control ... I really blew it ... What's the use of even trying anymore?* A sense of helplessness might set in, and you might not be able to summon up the energy to get back on your diet.

The dieters I work with are generally amazed when I tell them what I usually do at social events: I plan in advance to eat about 25 percent more calories—at most—than usual. Which is what I did last summer at my daughter's wedding. I skipped all the hors d'oeuvres except for a few raw vegetables. I ate all of my salad and part of the main course. I didn't eat any dessert. (I brought a lot of wedding cake home, though, and ate a small piece for my evening snack every night for the next week.) And do you know what? I had a fabulous time. I enjoyed what I ate and didn't feel deprived. In fact, I felt really good that I'd stuck to my plan and avoided overeating. The reason it was easy for me to do so? It's because of the idea I have: *Being thinner is more important to me than the momentary pleasure of overeating on special occasions.*

what are you thinking?

You might need to counter sabotaging thoughts many times while eating out or attending special events. You might feel disappointed that you can't eat whatever you feel like having. Use the following responses to prepare for sabotaging thoughts ahead of time.

Sabotaging Thought: I'm not the kind of person who can make special requests. I'm afraid that it will annoy the waiter.
Helpful Response: People make special requests all the time. I'm entitled to do so, too. Asking the waiter to modify my meal is okay. So is asking the waiter to wrap up leftovers for me to take home. If I were eating differently because I had a medical condition or a food allergy or because I was vegetarian, I wouldn't hesitate. Eating differently to lose weight is just as legitimate.

Sabotaging Thought: The food that's on my diet plan costs more than the food I really want to order. I can't justify spending more money just to stick to my diet.
Helpful Response: It's worth it! I'm worth it! What a great way to spend money— toward a goal that I really, really want to achieve.

Sabotaging Thought: My dining companions will notice that I'm eating differently from them (or from how I used to eat). They might say something that makes me feel uncomfortable.
Helpful Response: So what? If they comment, I can just say I'm trying to eat in a more healthy way. Then I can change the subject.

Sabotaging Thought: I wish I could eat what everyone else is eating.
Helpful Response: I also wish I were thinner. Oh, well. It's not fair, but it would be even less fair if I went ahead and ate what they were eating and, as a result, didn't lose weight.

Sabotaging Thought: This is a special occasion. I deserve to treat myself.
Helpful Response: If I want to lose weight and keep it off forever, I have to learn to celebrate in different ways. If I keep celebrating with food, I'll put myself at risk for gaining weight. It isn't worth it!

Sabotaging Thought: It's sad that I can't eat everything I want.
Helpful Response: It's SO WONDERFUL that I can stick with my plan and lose weight.

commit in writing

The next time I eat out, I'm going to: _____

_____

_____

_____

_____

_____

_____ .

> Once I start preparing myself in advance
> for eating out, dieting will be easier.

today's to-do list

Check off the tasks you've completed. For any item you haven't completed, record when you're going to complete it.

_____ I read my Advantages, NO CHOICE, It's Not Okay, and Get Back on Track Response Cards at least twice today.

_____ I read other Response Cards as needed.

_____ I ate slowly, sitting down and noticing every bite.

Circle one: Every time   Most of the time   Some of the time

_____ I gave myself credit for engaging in helpful eating behaviors.

Circle one: Every time   Most of the time   Some of the time

_____ I wrote a food plan for tomorrow and monitored everything I ate in writing right after I finished eating.

_____ I did spontaneous and planned exercise.

_____ I dealt effectively with issues of unfairness and discouragement.

_____ I decided how I'll respond to food pushers.

_____ I planned to eat out this week.

day 31

Decide About Drinking

Does your diet plan discourage alcohol? If so, how do you feel about giving it up? Drinking alcohol is an individual choice. My personal decision is to have a drink only occasionally because I'd *much* rather spend my calories on food.

If you want to fit drinking into your diet, you need to plan your alcohol intake in advance, just as you do your food intake. This means limiting your consumption and making sure that alcohol doesn't loosen your inhibitions about eating.

The Facts About Alcohol

Unfortunately, alcohol contains calories—a lot. At 7 calories a gram, it's nearly twice as caloric, gram for gram, as protein and carbohydrates (both of which are about 4 calories per gram). Plus, most of the mixers that go into alcoholic drinks are highly caloric. One mixed drink can easily contain 400 calories!

Many dieters try to make up for those calories by eating less. But eating less can lead you to eat more later. Plus, alcohol itself tends to lower your inhibitions, making you much more likely to overeat or eat something you hadn't planned.

You might think it's okay to make spontaneous decisions to drink. But just as you've had to learn to eliminate spontaneous eating and stick to your food plan, you have to learn to eliminate spontaneous drinking. Otherwise, you put yourself at risk, sooner or later, for gaining weight. You need to make decisions about whether and how much to drink today, before you find yourself presented with the question. Otherwise, you're likely to drink too much.

How Much, How Often

Think about your choices: You can decide not to drink at all, or you can set some kind of limit. For example, you might decide to have one drink a day, a week, a month, or somewhere in-between. Or you might have a drink just on special occasions. If you choose to drink, you'll need to figure out how to fit it in without taking in too many calories. Ask yourself, *Do I really want to spend my calories this way? Would I rather eat _____ or _____ instead?*

If you struggle with this decision, write out a list of the advantages and disadvantages of drinking and talk about your decision with your diet coach.

Come up with a plan that works for you. Margaret, for example, decided that she wouldn't drink at home, only when she was out with friends. Once she made this a firm rule, she had little difficulty giving up her nightly glass of wine. Ken, on the other hand, is a beer connoisseur. He decided that he'd drink only one beer a day, having it with dinner so he wouldn't be tempted to accompany his beer with any unplanned snacks.

Whatever you decide to do about alcohol is fine, as long as:

- You don't skimp on food.
- You plan when and how much you'll drink.
- You calculate beforehand how caloric the drink is.
- You don't allow alcohol to lead to unplanned eating.

what are you thinking?

Do you have unhelpful thoughts about limiting your drinking? If so, remind yourself that many people don't drink, even though they'd like to, because they're also watching their weight, have a health problem, have a drinking problem, or get unpleasant side effects from alcohol. You're not the only one who has to restrict or eliminate alcohol intake.

Sabotaging thoughts are common among people attempting to cut out or cut back on alcohol. Create Response Cards to combat any you think apply to you.

Sabotaging Thought: I feel like having a drink.
Helpful Response: I may feel like drinking, but that doesn't give me license to drink. I sometimes feel like buying things I can't afford or yelling at my boss, but I don't. I'd rather feel proud instead of guilty. I'd rather be thinner.

Sabotaging Thought: I can't have fun unless I drink as much as I want.
Helpful Response: It isn't all or nothing. I can still enjoy myself socially—like millions of other people who don't drink or don't drink much.

Sabotaging Thought: The people I'm with will think I'm no fun if I don't drink.
Helpful Response: That may or may not be true. What's more important to me, anyway: what they think or whether I'm doing what it takes to lose weight?

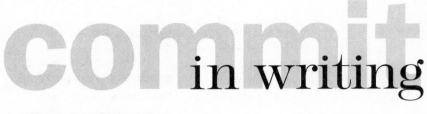

commit in writing

My decision about drinking is: _____

_____

_____

_____

_____

_____

_____ .

> Once I accept the fact that I need to limit
> my drinking, dieting will be easier.

today's to-do list

Check off the tasks you've completed. For any item you haven't completed, record when you're going to complete it.

_____ I read my Advantages, NO CHOICE, It's Not Okay, and Get Back on Track Response Cards at least twice today.

_____ I read other Response Cards as needed.

_____ I ate slowly, sitting down and noticing every bite.

Circle one: Every time   Most of the time   Some of the time

_____ I gave myself credit for engaging in helpful eating behaviors.

Circle one: Every time   Most of the time   Some of the time

_____ I wrote a food plan for tomorrow and monitored everything I ate in writing right after I finished eating.

_____ I did spontaneous and planned exercise.

_____ I dealt effectively with issues of unfairness and discouragement.

_____ I decided how much and how often I'll drink alcohol.

day 32
Prepare for Travel

Many dieters tell me that they feel anxious about gaining weight while on a trip. Teresa, for example, had been following a diet for several months and had lost a considerable amount of weight when the time came for her annual trip to the beach with her immediate and extended family. In past years, Teresa had gained an average of 4 to 5 pounds every time she went on vacation. She asked me, "How can I possibly follow my diet when I won't be in charge of the kitchen and when I'll be eating out a lot?"

I told her what I tell all dieters: Whether you're traveling for business or pleasure, you can stay in control if you plan a strategy before you go.

Making a Travel Plan

About a week before your trip, create a diet strategy. I want you to think about this in advance so that you can remind yourself of it every day before you leave. Decide how closely you'll follow your diet, specifically what exceptions you'll make and how much weight, if any, you'll allow yourself to gain. These decisions are individual. There are no right or wrong answers. Some people do better if they try to follow their diet as closely as possible when they're away, so that they don't gain any weight during this time. This strategy, however, is totally unrealistic for most people. If your eating rules are too strict, you might get fed up and abandon your diet altogether. A better strategy might be one of the following:

- Allow yourself a few hundred extra calories every day. (This is what I do.)
- Follow your usual plan every day but add minor splurges on a few occasions.
- Follow your diet every day except for a splurge on the last day.

Using any one of these strategies might cause a small weight gain (assuming your splurges aren't too big), which is reasonable and certainly much better than gaining a lot of weight. You'll feel better about yourself if you

If your eating rules are too strict, you might get fed up and abandon your diet altogether.

decide in advance that this is what you want to do. You won't feel very good if you try not to gain weight, eat more than you'd planned, and end up gaining weight anyway.

To figure out what your strategy should be, think about which foods or beverages you'll most want to have while you're away. Will you enjoy sipping mixed drinks at the bar? Indulging in a rich dessert after dinner? Sampling new and unusual foods?

Once you create your strategy, write it down in your diet notebook. Read it every day until you leave (and every day while you're there), so you'll have this strategy firmly in your mind.

How Not to Gain Too Much

Try to think of specific situations that might arise while you're away that will test your resolve. Then figure out what you'll do about them. Consult your diet coach, if you like.

These are some solutions dieters I've counseled use to help prevent gaining too much weight while they're away from home:

Exercise more. It will help counteract small amounts of overeating. You can either do formal exercise or take advantage of recreational activities that require a moderate to high expenditure of energy.

Eat brunch instead of breakfast and lunch. If you sleep later than usual, combining these two meals will allow you to eat a larger meal in one sitting.

Carry food with you. If you have a long trip ahead of you, consider bringing along some favorite foods permitted on your diet plan. While in transit, be careful not to eat out of boredom. Also beware of eating more meals than you had planned, due to time changes. Some dieters I work with ask their hotel in advance for a mini refrigerator (or they ask the management to remove the alcohol that is already in the minibar). When they arrive at their destination, they find a grocery store and buy some food and drinks, especially for planned snacks.

Use the strategies you've already learned. Take this book with you. Reread how to differentiate hunger from cravings and how to tolerate them; how to use anti-craving techniques; how to prepare for unplanned eating and overeating; how to get back on your diet after a slipup; how to handle disappointment and the unfairness issue; how to deal with food pushers; and, especially, how to prepare for eating out and drinking alcohol. You've learned a tremendous amount if you've been practicing the skills in this program for the last month. Use that knowledge!

During the Trip Home

You're on the way home. You tried to follow your predetermined diet plan while you were away. How did you do? You should be giving yourself credit for everything you did right. But maybe you slipped some. Are you dreading getting on the scale?

Tell yourself, *When I get on the scale, I might be heavier ... That's okay, I planned to gain a little weight ... As soon as I get home, I'll have more control over my food and my environment, and I'll lose it again.* Make your trip home your symbolic transition from vacation eating to dieting.

Plan what you're going to eat for the rest of the day as well as tomorrow. Many dieters try to quickly undo their weight gain by overly restricting their eating when they return. Avoid this temptation because it will put you at risk for overeating within a few days. Make sure to reestablish your helpful eating behaviors, such as eating everything slowly and while sitting down, planning your meals in writing the night before, and monitoring everything you eat. Also, call your diet coach as soon as you get home.

what are you thinking?

Vacations are ripe for sabotaging thoughts. Prepare for them now, so you can convincingly respond to them in the moment.

Sabotaging Thought: Oh, no, I won't have control over food while I'm on vacation. What if I gain a lot of weight?
Helpful Response: I've developed my vacation diet strategy. I'll get my diet notebook right now and read the plan.

Sabotaging Thought: I've been so good. I should be able to eat whatever I want while I'm away. If I can't eat whatever I want, I won't have any fun.
Helpful Response: It's not all or nothing. I won't have to deprive myself completely. I'll still be able to eat some foods I like. I won't be giving up all pleasure of eating, and I won't be giving up all fun. Besides, when I return home, I'll be happy when I step on the scale and realize I haven't gained 5 pounds. It will be worth it.

Sabotaging Thought: It's not fair that I can't eat whatever I want when I'm on vacation.
Helpful Response: That's true. It's not fair. But I can't have it both ways. I can't eat whatever I want without gaining a significant amount of weight. I've worked hard to lose weight so far. It's not worth it to eat uncontrollably and lose a lot of ground.

commit in writing

My vacation diet strategy will be: _____
_____
_____
_____
_____
_____
_____
_____ .

Once I accept that I have to follow
through with my vacation diet strategy,
dieting will be easier.

today's to-do list

Check off the tasks you've completed. For any item you haven't completed, record when you're going to complete it.

_____ I read my Advantages, NO CHOICE, It's Not Okay, and Get Back on Track Response Cards at least twice today.

_____ I read other Response Cards as needed.

_____ I ate slowly, sitting down and noticing every bite.

Circle one: Every time   Most of the time   Some of the time

_____ I gave myself credit for engaging in helpful eating behaviors.

Circle one: Every time   Most of the time   Some of the time

_____ I wrote a food plan for tomorrow and monitored everything I ate in writing right after I finished eating.

_____ I did spontaneous and planned exercise.

_____ I planned how I'll eat when I travel.

day 33

Eliminate Emotional Eating

Just about everyone with a weight problem eats for emotional reasons from time to time. One dieter I worked with, Pam, ate when she was anxious or sad. Patricia ate when she felt overwhelmed. Robert ate when he was lonely or bored. Lucy ate when she was angry.

Like these dieters, you might soothe yourself with food because you don't like feeling distressed or bored. Food can certainly be an effective distractor—temporarily. But eating doesn't solve the problem that led to your distress in the first place. In fact, eating emotionally creates another problem: You feel bad about straying from your diet.

Ella often ate when she was out of sorts. For example, one day, Ella's boss asked her to stay late at work for a third night in a row. Ella had many negative thoughts: *He is so inconsiderate! Doesn't he think I have a life? Why should I have to work late? Why doesn't he ask someone else?* These thoughts left her fuming. When she got home late, she was still upset and completely abandoned her food plan. When she'd finished polishing off a pint of ice cream, she got mad at herself.

Had Ella been able to look at the situation more dispassionately, she might have been able to do some problem solving. She might have realized that she could have nicely, but assertively, turned down her boss's request. But even if there wasn't a good solution to the problem, she didn't need to eat. She could have responded to her angry thoughts and decreased her distress. Instead, she got riled up, couldn't stand feeling that way, and tried to soothe herself with food.

Contrast Ella's behavior with that of people without weight problems. It would never occur to most of them to eat when they were upset. They don't rely on food to help them feel better.

> ## People without a weight problem
> ### *don't think of eating to feel better.*

How to Calm Down

There is nothing wrong with having negative emotions. They're just nature's way of telling us there's a problem. Do you think that you can't tolerate negative emotions? You can! Of course, you don't like feeling upset. But negative emotions aren't dangerous. Nothing bad will happen to you. You won't fall apart. Given enough time, negative emotions—just like cravings—will subside on their own. You don't have to eat. A negative emotion is not an emergency.

> Food can be an effective distractor—temporarily. But *eating doesn't solve the problem that led to your distress* in the first place.

But negative emotions are uncomfortable, and there are Cognitive Therapy strategies you can learn to feel better. Usually, the best way to decrease your distress is to respond to your negative thinking and to solve the problem associated with your emotional upset. You'll learn how to do this tomorrow. But it's sometimes difficult to go right to problem solving (and there might be some problems that are out of your control), especially if you're accustomed to immediately reaching for food when you're upset. You might need to decrease your distress first, in non-food-related ways.

Fortunately, you've already developed many of the skills you'll need for dealing with emotional eating. You'll use the same techniques learned on pages 121–134 to tolerate the unpleasant sensations of hunger and craving and to decrease your urges to eat. Read on to discover how to do this.

Use Mindset Techniques
Apply the same kind of thinking techniques you previously learned to combat emotional eating:

Label how you're feeling. Tell yourself, *I'm just feeling upset ... I'm not hungry.*

Stand firm. Tell yourself you're absolutely *not* going to eat just because you're distressed. Remind yourself that you don't want to strengthen your giving-in muscle and weaken your resistance muscle by straying from your food plan. Think about how eating at this point will undermine your confidence in your ability to stick with your diet.

Don't give yourself a choice. Once you say to yourself with conviction, *NO CHOICE ... I'm definitely not going to eat,* you'll stop struggling. You *will* struggle, though, if you waver and say to yourself, *I hate feeling like this ... I don't know if I can stand not eating.*

Imagine the aftermath of giving in. Visualize eating. How long does the pleasure of eating really last? Now, imagine the rest of the picture.

do you eat emotionally?

Emotional eating involves a desire to distract yourself from an unpleasant feeling. When you find yourself eating for a reason other than true hunger, ask yourself, *How was I just feeling emotionally?*

- *Was I feeling sad, lonely, worried, embarrassed, frustrated, angry, guilty?*
- *Was I feeling at loose ends, unsettled, bored?*
- *Was I trying to avoid doing something I didn't want to do?*

Remind yourself of how many times in your life (dozens? hundreds? more?) you promised yourself you weren't going to stray from a diet. See yourself getting more and more heavy-hearted, discouraged, disappointed in yourself. See how bad you feel that you gave in. Pause for a moment. Now that you've seen the whole picture, which seems better: eating or not eating?

Read your Advantages Response Card. Review all the reasons you want to lose weight. Don't you still want to achieve all those benefits? Aren't they still important? Is it worth strengthening your giving-in muscle by eating now?

> ## *You have to deal with distress in non-food-related ways* if you want to sustain permanent weight loss.

Most important, remind yourself that you simply will not be able to sustain weight loss if you continue to eat for emotional reasons. You must learn different ways of handling distress so you don't turn to food for comfort.

Use Behavioral Techniques

Take some action in order to decrease your distress when you're upset:

Distract yourself. When you're upset, watching TV or reading might not be distracting enough. Look at My Distraction Activities Chart on page 132 to choose a few activities to try.

Drink a soothing no- or low-calorie beverage. Consider making yourself a cup of tea. Sit down and drink it slowly.

Relax. Listen to an audiotape that teaches relaxation techniques, such as progressive muscle relaxation, guided imagery, or deep breathing. Or do the slow, shallow breathing described on page 131.

The more you practice these mindset and behavioral techniques, the better you'll get at them. Initially, you'll find that the techniques are more effective when you're experiencing mild to moderate levels of negative emotions. As you become more proficient, you'll also be able to use them when you experience more intense emotions.

Apply several of these techniques as soon as you start to feel upset. Once you calm down, work on solving the problem that led to the negative emotion in the first place. (I'll be addressing this tomorrow.) Instead of saying to yourself, *If I'm upset, I'll deal with it by eating,* tell yourself, *If I'm upset, I'll try to solve the problem ... If I can't focus on problem solving, I can use my mindset and behavioral tools first.*

what are you thinking?

Do you feel unsure about your ability to get control of emotional eating? If so, take a moment to identify and respond to your sabotaging thoughts.

Sabotaging Thought: I can't calm down without eating.
Helpful Response: There are lots of techniques I can use instead of turning to food. I'll be very glad in a little while that I didn't compound the original problem by eating.

Sabotaging Thought: I deserve to eat when I'm feeling bad.
Helpful Response: I deserve to feel better. I deserve comfort. But I also deserve to be thinner. Comforting myself with food will only work temporarily, and I'll feel even worse later.

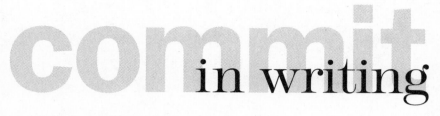

commit in writing

The next time I'm upset, I'm going to: _____

_____

_____

_____

_____ .

Once I start using strategies
other than eating to calm down,
dieting will be easier.

today's to-do list

Check off the tasks you've completed. For any item you haven't completed, record when you're going to complete it.

_____ I read my Advantages, NO CHOICE, It's Not Okay, and Get Back on Track Response Cards at least twice today.

_____ I read other Response Cards as needed.

_____ I ate slowly, sitting down and noticing every bite.

Circle one: Every time   Most of the time   Some of the time

_____ I gave myself credit for engaging in helpful eating behaviors.

Circle one: Every time   Most of the time   Some of the time

_____ I wrote a food plan for tomorrow and monitored everything I ate in writing right after I finished eating.

_____ I did spontaneous and planned exercise.

_____ I planned how I'll handle negative emotions without eating.

day 34

Solve Problems

Today, you're going to learn how to become a more effective problem solver. Thinking clearly about a problem, even if you haven't figured out a solution, can help you feel more in control, less upset, and, therefore, less likely to turn to emotional eating.

Identify the Problem

To solve a problem, you first have to define it. Sometimes, this is easy: Perhaps your boss put a lot of pressure on you, you bounced a check, or someone made a negative comment about you. Sometimes, the problem isn't so easy to pinpoint. You might notice the emotion but not feel sure about what led to it. Consider asking a friend or your diet coach to help you sort things through.

Once you've defined the problem, be sure to identify the negative thoughts running through your mind. Then use the Seven Question Technique to respond to your negative thoughts. Think about the following that you learned on Day 27 (pages 199–203):

1. What kind of thinking error could I be making? (See Day 26 on pages 195–198 for help.)
2. What evidence is there that this thought might not be true or might not be completely true?
3. Is there an alternative explanation or another way of viewing this?
4. What is the most realistic outcome of this situation?
5. What is the effect of my believing this negative thought and what could be the effect of changing my thinking?
6. What would I tell my friend if she were in this situation and had this same kind of thought?
7. What should I do now?

"What should I do now?" will help you solve the problem. Think of various solutions. Weigh the pros and cons of each. Pick one solution to try and see how it works, just like Dena, a dieter I counseled, did.

Tired from a full day of work and from all of her mom responsibilities, Dena would invariably flop on the couch and begin thinking of all of the chores she still had to do. The thought, *I'll never get everything done that I need to,* led to her feeling anxious. To decrease her anxiety without eating, Dena used the Seven Question Technique, as shown on the facing page.

1. What kind of thinking error could I be making?
Fortune telling
2. What evidence is there that this thought might not be true or not completely true?
I've had this thought in the past, and somehow I always get the most important things done.
3. Is there an alternative explanation or another way of viewing this?
Maybe I shouldn't even try to get everything done tonight.
4. What is the most realistic outcome of this situation?
That I'll be able to get some things done but not everything. I'll have to do the rest another time.
5. What is the effect of my believing this negative thought? What could be the effect of changing my thinking?
I feel really overwhelmed and paralyzed. If I changed my thinking, I'd feel less anxious and could get started on doing something sooner.
6. What would I tell my friend if she were in this situation and had this thought?
I'd tell her to get up right away and do whatever seems easiest, like putting a load of laundry in the washing machine. Then do whatever else seems relatively easy—cleaning the dishes, taking out the trash, whatever.
7. What should I do now?
Start right now with a load of laundry and then call Jennifer for support.

You Can't Solve Every Problem

You also need to be realistic. There are some things that may be beyond your control. Your partner could have an alcohol problem. You could have a serious health condition. You're likely to be *very* upset. What can you do?

First, you *should* feel bad about these kinds of things. You wouldn't be human if you weren't upset. If you're drawing an unrealistic conclusion about these real-life problems, however, you might be able to respond to your negative thinking. For example, you might have the thought, *Because of this problem, I'm going to have a miserable life.* The Seven Question Technique might be useful in this circumstance.

Whether or not you've drawn unrealistic conclusions, though, make sure to seek support. You need to talk to other people. Ask them to listen. Tell them what they can do to help in practical ways. For example, they might have some ideas of what you can do to make your life better, given these uncontrollable circumstances. If you find that you're still having a hard time dealing with your feelings, consider seeking help from a mental-health professional or spiritual advisor. Reach out.

what are you thinking?

As you work on solving problems, many sabotaging thoughts can get in your way, undermining your confidence and leading you to automatically discount potential solutions. Use the following examples to help you respond to these thoughts.

Sabotaging Thought: I can't do this. I can't solve this problem.
Helpful Response: Most problems can be solved—or partially solved—even if I don't see the solution right now.

Sabotaging Thought: This solution isn't going to work.
Helpful Response: It might or might not. Maybe I should try it. I can call on a friend to help me figure out what to do.

Sabotaging Thought: I don't even want to think about the problem. I'd rather just eat.
Helpful Response: Eating is just a short-term fix that'll make me feel even worse in the long run.

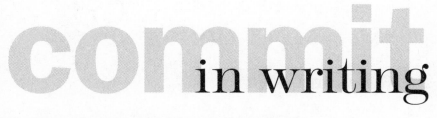

commit in writing

The next time I have a problem, instead of turning to food, I'll: _____

_____

_____

_____

_____ .

Once you recognize that food
won't make your problems go away,
dieting will be easier.

today's to-do list

Check off the tasks you've completed. For any item you haven't completed, record when you're going to complete it.

_____ I read my Advantages, NO CHOICE, It's Not Okay, and Get Back on Track Response Cards at least twice today.

_____ I read other Response Cards as needed.

_____ I ate slowly, sitting down and noticing every bite.

Circle one: Every time   Most of the time   Some of the time

_____ I gave myself credit for engaging in helpful eating behaviors.

Circle one: Every time   Most of the time   Some of the time

_____ I wrote a food plan for tomorrow and monitored everything I ate in writing right after I finished eating.

_____ I did spontaneous and planned exercise.

_____ I reminded myself how I plan to handle negative emotions without eating.

_____ I resolved to use the Seven Question Technique the next time I'm upset instead of turning to food for comfort.

day 35
Get Ready to Weigh In

Tomorrow marks the end of your fifth week using the Beck Diet Solution. If you've been following all the steps in this book, chances are good that you'll see a lower weight tomorrow.

Before you step on the scale in the morning, remember that whatever number it shows is just information. If you're nervous or expect that you've gained weight, reread Day 28 (pages 204–205) before you weigh yourself.

After you weigh yourself, calculate the change in your weight, place a dot on the weight-loss graph, and connect the dots. Contact your diet coach to tell him or her how much your weight changed. If you've lost a half pound or more, great! If you haven't, don't get discouraged. Just remember to review your eating plan with your diet coach if it turns out that you've stayed the same weight or gained weight for two weeks in a row.

Consider carrying your weight-loss graph around with you to look at every so often to remind yourself of your progress. One dieter I worked with made a miniature version of her weight-loss graph on the back of a business card that she saw every time she opened her wallet. Looking at the graph made her think these positive thoughts to herself: *Look what I've done! I love how the line on this graph keeps going down! I'm so proud of myself! It's totally worth everything I'm doing.*

what are you thinking?

Your sabotaging thoughts about weighing in might be similar to the thoughts you had about your weigh-in last week. Here's another sabotaging thought that might surface tomorrow.

Sabotaging Thought: I know it's reasonable to have lost only a half pound this week, but I'm still disappointed.

Helpful Response: My weight is going down. That's good! It means that what I've been doing is working. I should celebrate each and every half-pound weight loss. If I hope for something unrealistic, I'll be disappointed. I'm going in the right direction. That's what counts. I really deserve a lot of credit for using the mindset and behavioral techniques I've learned and for weighing less than I did when I started this program.

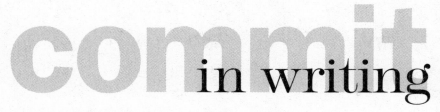

commit in writing

Before I step on the scale tomorrow, I'm going to remind myself: _____

_____

_____

_____.

Once I develop realistic expectations
for weight loss, dieting will be easier.

today's to-do list

Check off the tasks you've completed. For any item you haven't completed, record when you're going to complete it.

_____ I read my Advantages, NO CHOICE, It's Not Okay, and Get Back on Track Response Cards at least twice today.

_____ I read other Response Cards as needed.

_____ I ate slowly, sitting down and noticing every bite.

Circle one: Every time   Most of the time   Some of the time

_____ I gave myself credit for engaging in helpful eating behaviors.

Circle one: Every time   Most of the time   Some of the time

_____ I wrote a food plan for tomorrow and monitored everything I ate in writing right after I finished eating.

_____ I did spontaneous and planned exercise.

_____ I reminded myself how I plan to handle negative emotions without eating.

_____ I resolved to use the Seven Question Technique when I'm upset instead of turning to food for comfort.

_____ I prepared for my weigh-in tomorrow.

chapter 10

Week 6

Fine-Tune Your New Skills

Congratulations on completing the first five weeks of the Beck Diet Solution. You've come a long way! Now you know what to do when you want to eat but you know you shouldn't. You've demonstrated over and over that you can take control of your eating. You can decide what's in your best interest to eat—and not eat—and how to get yourself to follow through with your food plans, even if you're hungry, craving, seeking comfort, being pressured to eat, or just tempted by food.

This week, you'll continue to fine-tune your Cognitive Therapy skills. You'll learn how to continue to build your confidence by recognizing that you've lost weight due to your own efforts, using the new behavioral and mindset techniques you've acquired. You'll learn how to reduce your overall stress so that you can continue to have time and energy for dieting. You'll learn what to do when your weight plateaus and how to keep up with exercise. You'll take steps toward enriching your life now—instead of waiting until you lose weight.

Finally, you'll develop a reminder system that will help you continue to use your strategies for a very long time. You'll improve your confidence, decrease stress, and enrich your life, so you'll reduce your risk of relapse and increase your chances of lasting success.

day 36
Believe It

When Brenda came to see me, she had more than 125 pounds she wanted to lose—and was convinced that she'd never be able to lose it. After all, despite the fact that she had "been on a diet" for 35 years, she was still growing heavier rather than lighter. She felt doomed to endlessly repeat her cycle of crash dieting, followed by out-of-control eating.

"I'm just not the kind of person who can lose weight," she told me. She continued to be skeptical that I could help her, even after I described the mindset and behavioral strategies I'd teach her. But Brenda said that she was willing to try.

As the weeks went by, Brenda slowly but steadily lost weight—but she remained skeptical. After she lost 10 pounds, she said, "It won't last." After she lost 20 pounds, she was confused: "I know the scale says I've lost this much weight, and I know my clothes are looser, but it just doesn't seem real." After she lost 30 pounds, she was very confused. The evidence that she was successfully losing weight was undeniable, but Brenda still doubted herself. "Okay, I *know* I've lost weight, but I don't know how I did it," she said. "It's just a fluke." After she lost a total of 40 pounds, she thought she had the answer: "I'm 40 pounds lighter, but that's only because you're helping me."

I reminded Brenda that although I certainly had been teaching her the Cognitive Therapy skills, *she* was the one who was consistently using them. *That's* why she was successfully losing weight. She understood this intellectually, but, on a deeper level, this just didn't fit with her view of herself as a person who couldn't lose weight.

For Brenda to keep making progress, I knew it was important for her to stop doubting herself. You might need to do so, too. Now five weeks into this program, you might be at the point most dieters eventually reach—the point where you question whether or not you can keep losing weight. At some point, you might say to yourself, *This is just a fluke ... I'll wake up tomorrow and I'll have gained it all back ... I'm no different from how I was the last time I tried to diet.*

But you *are* different. You now have critical skills that you didn't have in the past, and you've learned how to use them consistently and successfully. Your weight loss is not a fluke. Your progress won't disappear *as long as you continue to use your tools.*

To help change her perception of herself from someone who can't lose weight to someone who *can* lose weight, Brenda read the Response Card below every day for weeks. Use it for inspiration in creating your own card:

Believe It!

I'm losing weight because I've learned how. I now know:

1. What I have to do (e.g., plan my eating, eat slowly while sitting down, use anti-craving strategies)
2. What I have to remind myself (e.g., hunger and cravings are never emergencies, NO CHOICE, *Oh, well*)
3. How to motivate myself (get support, read my Advantages Response Card, give myself credit every day)
4. How to keep honest (report my weight change to my diet coach weekly)

Build More Confidence

Remind yourself what you were like five weeks ago, *before* you started this program. If that's hard to do, picture yourself during a holiday or special event that occurred around that time. In particular, take a look at the changes in your *behavior*. Before you started this program:

- How often did you eat standing up?
- How often did you eat mindlessly?
- How often did you eat too quickly?
- How often did you plan ahead of time what you were going to eat?
- How often did you overeat or eat for emotional reasons?
- How often did you criticize yourself (and become demoralized) for what you ate?

How often do you do these things anymore? Now, take a look at the changes in your *thinking*. Before you started this program:

- How often did you fool yourself? *(It won't matter if I overeat once. Calories don't count if I eat crumbs. I can't have a good time if I don't eat what I want. It's okay to eat this because I'm upset. I've strayed, so I may as well blow it for the day.)*
- How often did you dwell on injustice? *(It's not fair that I can't eat like other people. It's not fair that I can't eat whatever I want. It's not fair that I have to diet.)*
- How often did you let your concerns about other people stand in the way of doing what you needed to do for yourself? *(I can't inconvenience others. I have to keep them happy. I can't turn down food they offer me.)*

How often do you have these kinds of thoughts now and how do you respond to them when they do arise?

It's important to continually take stock of what you've learned and the progress you've made. You need to recognize that you've lost weight because of your own efforts. You can continue to make this happen. Reinforce this idea by writing in your diet notebook exactly how you're different, as Brenda did.

Below is what Brenda wrote in her diet notebook to remind herself of how far she'd come. She added to this list over time. Whenever she had a crisis of confidence, she would read it over to remind herself just how much she had changed.

Before I started this program, I couldn't consistently:

Leave food on my plate.
Feel hungry and not stress about it.
Say to myself, NO CHOICE.
Stop eating when I'd finished what was on my plate.
Make exercise a priority.
Stick to my plan.
Refrain from spontaneous eating.
Stop myself from nibbling at my dinner plate on the way to
   the table.
Eat slowly.
Eat sitting down.
Recognize and respond to my sabotaging thoughts.
Give myself credit.
Limit myself when I ate out.
Be assertive with food pushers.
Put myself first so I could eat properly.

what are you thinking?

Are you like Brenda? Do you sometimes doubt your ability to keep making progress? If so, it's important to respond to your sabotaging thoughts. Perhaps they're similar to some of these. Create Response Cards for any you think you might need.

Sabotaging Thought: If I start to believe that I can do this, I'll jinx myself.
Helpful Response: On the contrary, if I believe I can't do this, then I'm likely to run into trouble when dieting gets tougher. If I build up my confidence, I'll be able to keep plugging away.

Sabotaging Thought: If I recognize my progress, I'll get too confident and start to loosen up.
Helpful Response: I'll be able to catch myself, as long as I fill out the to-do lists every day.

commit in writing

Whenever I begin to worry that I can't lose weight, I'll tell myself: _____

_____

_____

_____

_____

_____

_____

_____

_____

_____

_____.

> Once I believe that I've
> lost weight due to my own efforts,
> dieting will be easier.

today's to-do list

Let's follow up on your efforts from previous weeks. Are you still doing the following:

- Consulting your diet coach
- Making dieting a priority
- Being assertive with others
- Tolerating hunger and cravings
- Responding to sabotaging thoughts

Check off the tasks you've completed. For any item you haven't completed, record when you're going to complete it.

_____ I read my Advantages, NO CHOICE, It's Not Okay, and Get Back on Track Response Cards at least twice today.

_____ I read other Response Cards as needed.

_____ I ate slowly, sitting down and noticing every bite.

Circle one: Every time   Most of the time   Some of the time

_____ I gave myself credit for engaging in helpful eating behaviors.

Circle one: Every time   Most of the time   Some of the time

_____ I wrote a food plan for tomorrow and monitored everything I ate in writing right after I finished eating.

_____ I did spontaneous and planned exercise.

_____ I created a Believe It! Response Card to build my confidence.

_____ I wrote a progress report in my diet notebook.

_____ I reminded myself of all of the new behavioral and mindset changes I've made during the last five weeks.

_____ I weighed myself, recorded the results on my weight-loss graph, and reported my change in weight to my diet coach.

day 37

Reduce Stress

Everyone experiences some type of stress every day. In fact, mild stress can actually be helpful if it motivates you to be productive. But moderate to high levels of stress are counterproductive. Even if you're not under much stress today, you will be sooner or later, so prepare yourself now.

Three Steps to Lower Your Level of Stress

On Days 33 and 34 (pages 227–235) of this program, you learned how to cope with negative emotions and to solve problems that cause them. You'll use many of the same skills to cope with problems that create stress. Here are the steps you should take:

Step 1: Solve the Problem

If you're stressed because you have too many demands or responsibilities, go back to My Priority Chart (page 104) and divide your activities into essential, highly desirable, and desirable categories. Use the Seven Question Technique (pages 199–203) to respond to negative thoughts that interfere with problem solving. You might also find it helpful to ask a friend or your diet coach for help.

Step 2: Relax

Chronic stress can make your body tense. Consider getting an audiotape that teaches relaxation techniques, such as progressive muscle relaxation or guided imagery. Slow, controlled breathing, which I discussed earlier on page 131, should also help.

Step 3: Change Your Mindset

Many people are chronically stressed because they allow unreasonable rules to guide their behavior. These rules usually have the word *should* or *shouldn't* in them. Do any of the following sound familiar?

- *I should always do my best.*
- *I should always prevent problems from happening.*
- *I shouldn't rely on others.*
- *I shouldn't let people down.*
- *I shouldn't make others unhappy.*

Lillian, for example, has a rule: *I should always put other people first.* Therefore, even though it was the busiest time of the year at work, she agreed to help her mother buy a new computer, go with a friend to a concert, and help her cousin with gardening. Michael has an unspoken rule: *I can't show any sign of weakness.* Therefore, he didn't take time off from work when he had the flu (and it took him longer to recover). Suzanne also has a rule: *I should do everything myself.* Therefore, she deprived herself of the assistance she needed when her husband's chronic illness took a turn for the worse.

To reduce stress, you have to change your rules. Here's how:

Identify the rules you have for yourself. Your "shoulds" and "shouldn'ts" will probably show up when you try to do problem solving, and you'll exclude reasonable solutions if your rules are too rigid.

Gail was stressed at work. She knew the logical solution was to delegate some responsibilities. When she thought of doing so, though, her rule surfaced: *I shouldn't let others do anything important because they might screw it up.*

Catherine was stressed from being home with two toddlers. She needed time for herself, but her rule—*I shouldn't ask others for help*—interfered.

Relax your self-imposed rules. Use these suggestions to change them:

- Think of someone with more relaxed standards. What rules does he or she go by?
- Consider whether you would want your loved ones to live by a particular rule. Can you see how it would lead to stress? What rule would you rather they have for themselves?
- Think of the advantages of changing your rules.
- Take the words *always* and *never* out of your rules.
- Insert the word *reasonable* into your rules:
  - —*I should always do my best* becomes *I should try to do a reasonable job most of the time.*
  - —*I should always prevent problems from happening* becomes *I should try to take reasonable precautions.*
  - —*I shouldn't ever rely on others* becomes *I should rely on others when it is reasonable to do so.*

Relax your rules for others. You'll also be stressed if you have unreasonable expectations of other people. Do you believe:

- Other people should always be perfect?
- Other people should be able to read your mind?
- Other people should always be grateful?
- Other people shouldn't make you unhappy?
- Other people shouldn't treat you unfairly?
- Other people shouldn't misunderstand you?

Jackie, for example, was annoyed with customers who complained to her about the quality of her company's service: *They shouldn't take it out on me!* James was resentful that his neighbors didn't reach out to him: *They should be nicer.* Jill was worried because she thought others were too irresponsible: *They should be much more careful.*

Your "shoulds" and "shouldn'ts" show up when you have unrealistic rules about the way other people behave. When Tom was annoyed with his teenagers, he looked at his rules for them: *They should be more appreciative. They should help around the house more.* Bobbie was unhappy with her family because of her rule: *People should give back to me as much as I give to them.*

To relax your rules for other people, do the following:

- Recognize that you just don't have control—or not much control—over other people. The only one you really have control over is yourself. You can change your own thinking and behavior, but you can't necessarily change other people.
- Think about someone you admire who has more relaxed ideas about how others should be. What rules does he or she have?
- Think of the advantages of changing your rules.
- Try to take the words *always* and *never* out of your rules.
- Change "should" or "shouldn't" to "It's realistic to expect that...."
  —*Other people should always be perfect* becomes *It's realistic to expect that other people will make mistakes.*
  —*Other people should always read my mind* becomes *It's realistic to expect that people won't know what I want or need unless I tell them.*
  —*Other people should always be grateful* becomes *It's realistic to expect that not everyone will be as appreciative as I'd like them to be.*

what are you thinking?

As you think about the rules you have for yourself and others, you may feel resistant to change. If so, you probably have sabotaging thoughts that you need to address.

Sabotaging Thought: I've had these rules forever. How can I change them?
Helpful Response: I now have the skills to analyze my rules and ideas differently. I can also decide what is reasonable to do on a case-by-case basis.

Sabotaging Thought: If I lower my expectations for myself, I'll become completely unmotivated.
Helpful Response: It's not all or nothing. I don't have to lower my expectations completely, just enough to reduce my stress.

commit in writing

When I notice myself feeling stressed, I'll: _____

_____

_____

_____

_____

_____

_____ .

Once I take steps to reduce my overall stress, dieting will be easier.

today's to-do list

Check off the tasks you've completed. For any item you haven't completed, record when you're going to complete it.

_____ I read my Advantages, NO CHOICE, It's Not Okay, Get Back on Track, and Believe It! Response Cards at least twice today.

_____ I read other Response Cards as needed.

_____ I ate slowly, sitting down and noticing every bite.

Circle one: Every time   Most of the time   Some of the time

_____ I gave myself credit for engaging in helpful eating behaviors.

Circle one: Every time   Most of the time   Some of the time

_____ I wrote a food plan for tomorrow and monitored everything I ate in writing right after I finished eating.

_____ I did spontaneous and planned exercise.

_____ I worked toward changing my unreasonable rules for myself and others.

_____ I planned how I'll reduce stress.

day 38

Deal with a Plateau

Many dieters think that they should be able to lose weight every week without interruption. Do you think so, too? Let me ask you this: Has that been your experience in the past? Most people lose some weight, stay the same for a week or two, lose some more, gain a little back, lose some more, plateau for a week or two, and so on.

Some plateaus are short-lived. You might step on the scale one week and see no weight loss, but the next week you do. These mini plateaus are normal. They might be due to water retention, hormonal changes, or other biological influences. Or maybe you took in too many calories that week or exercised too little. Occasional plateaus and small weight gains are inevitable.

If you expect the scale to go down every week, you're setting yourself up for disappointment. As time goes on, you might find that you plateau for several weeks in a row. A number of studies have determined that nearly all dieters with a significant amount of weight to lose (more than 20 pounds) hit a plateau within the first six months of dieting.

Today, I'm not talking about short-lived plateaus. I'm talking about more lengthy plateaus that span a few weeks or longer. The most likely explanation for these plateaus is that your body no longer needs as much energy (calories) as you've been taking in. If you hit one of these longer plateaus, you have four options:

1. Continue to do what you're doing and see if you start to lose weight again.
2. Reduce your daily calorie intake by 200 calories, which should allow you to lose about a half pound per week. (Check with your health-care professional first to make sure it's reasonable to cut down some more.)
3. Increase your daily exercise by 15 to 20 minutes.
4. Call this your goal weight and move into maintenance.

You should expect occasional weight gains or plateaus, even if you've been doing everything right.

what are you thinking?

You might not have the following thoughts today, but they'll likely surface when you actually reach a plateau. Use them to create Response Cards so you'll have them ready when you need them.

Sabotaging Thought: It's terrible that I've hit a plateau.

Helpful Response: Reaching a plateau is a normal part of losing weight. I'm feeling discouraged now because I put in a lot of effort. But this is supposed to happen from time to time. It doesn't necessarily mean I'm doing anything wrong. I can ask my diet coach for help.

Sabotaging Thought: This just isn't fair. I've really worked hard. I should keep losing, like I have up until this point.

Helpful Response: I have a choice now. I can dwell on how unfair it seems that the scale didn't go lower. Or I can focus on how much weight I've lost up to this point and give myself credit for all of the changes I've made in my thinking and behavior so far.

commit in writing

When I reach a plateau, I'll: _____
_____
_____
_____
_____
_____
_____
_____.

Once I accept that plateaus are
normal, dieting will be easier.

today's to-do list

Check off the tasks you've completed. For any item you haven't completed, record when you're going to complete it.

_____ I read my Advantages, NO CHOICE, It's Not Okay, Get Back on Track, and Believe It! Response Cards at least twice today.

_____ I read other Response Cards as needed.

_____ I ate slowly, sitting down and noticing every bite.

Circle one: Every time   Most of the time   Some of the time

_____ I gave myself credit for engaging in helpful eating behaviors.

Circle one: Every time   Most of the time   Some of the time

_____ I wrote a food plan for tomorrow and monitored everything I ate in writing right after I finished eating.

_____ I did spontaneous and planned exercise.

_____ I planned what I'll do when I reach a plateau.

day 39
Keep Up with Exercise

When Claire came to see me, she was, as she put it, "completely out of shape." She had a sedentary job. Her favorite hobbies were watching TV, surfing the Internet, and reading. She didn't like to play sports—never had. She told me that she knew for certain she just wasn't an exercise person. She said she was pretty weak, and she could never physically exert herself like other people. To compound matters, her stamina was very low and she suffered from back pain intermittently.

As I do with all dieters I counsel, I told Claire about the benefits of exercise and suggested she start with just 10 to 15 minutes a day. She resisted, asking, "Can't I lose weight without exercising?" I continued to discuss with her the research about exercise and weight loss and maintenance. She grudgingly agreed to try walking for 10 to 15 minutes, at least four times a week.

When Claire returned for her next session, she reported that she'd walked four times but that she didn't like it. When I asked her what had gone through her mind before she left for her walks, she said, "I was thinking, *I really, really don't want to go ... I'd rather stay home and watch TV.*" During her walks, she had more sabotaging thoughts, such as, *This is boring ... Why do I have to do this?* After her walks, she'd say negative things to herself: *I didn't like that. Besides, it was just a drop in the bucket! What good is 10 minutes of exercise? I don't want to keep on doing it.*

No wonder Claire had never exercised consistently in the past! Her sabotaging thoughts kept getting in her way.

Like Claire, you might also resist exercise, because you don't like it, you're too busy or stressed, or you have a physical problem. You know the benefits of both planned and spontaneous exercise, but are you still exercising? Have you, over time, increased the amount of exercise? Is exercising still near the top of your priority list? Do you have a positive attitude toward exercise?

If you answered no to any of those questions, you'll need to respond to your sabotaging thoughts and solve some problems. How can you turn things around? You can do what Claire did.

Use the same techniques to motivate yourself to exercise that you used to motivate yourself to diet.

How Claire Changed

To encourage herself to exercise, Claire did the following:

- She asked her next-door neighbor to walk with her twice a week.
- She got books on tape from the library and downloaded music and podcasts to listen to when she walked on the treadmill or at a nearby park.
- She called her best friend on her cell phone while she was walking.
- She went back to reading her Response Cards before she started walking to remind herself of the benefits of losing weight that she'd listed at the beginning of the diet, as well as the benefits of exercise (see Day 9 on pages 107–112).
- She read a Response Card after she exercised, one that reminded her why she deserved so much credit for walking.

These strategies were enough to get Claire to walk at least three days a week, but still not enough to get her to do so with a wholly positive attitude. Then something happened: Claire hurt her back. The pain was severe enough that she had to go to a doctor who, after Claire had recovered to some degree, insisted that she get physical therapy. Although she was quite intimidated at the prospect, she was motivated to feel better and to stay free of pain. So she started going. Her physical therapist started her off slowly. He was encouraging and supportive. Claire began to do the recommended stretches at home between sessions, and her back slowly healed. She was proud of herself for making herself go to her appointments and for doing her daily exercises at home. She actually began to feel good before, during, and after exercising. She began to change her view of herself: *Maybe I can do this. I am getting stronger.*

When Claire's back healed, her physical therapist recommended that she go to a gym. Claire discussed the possibility with me, saying, "I know it's a good idea. But I'm just too intimidated." I reminded Claire that she had the same reluctance when she first started going to physical therapy. Claire took my suggestion to visit a nearby gym to see what it was like. The staff was friendly, very few people were model thin, and the whole experience was much less intimidating than she had predicted. She also talked to a personal trainer while she was there about the possibility of signing up for a few sessions.

With significant trepidation, Claire signed up. Since her birthday was the following week, she told everyone in her family that she wanted sessions with a personal trainer as a birthday present. It was difficult for her to make herself go at first, but she kept all her appointments. Her trainer was so encouraging that she left each session thinking, *Hey, that was good,* instead of her usual, *I didn't like that ... I wish I didn't have to do it.*

After a few weeks, Claire started to get a sense of mastery. Soon she felt comfortable enough to stop working with a personal trainer and start working out on her own. She transformed her view of herself from a person who "knew" she was weak, had no stamina, and was incapable of sustaining an exercise program, to a person who kept getting stronger and stronger and knew for sure she would keep it up for life.

How You Can Change

Is there something that stops you from getting consistent exercise? Like Claire, do you view yourself as a non-exerciser? Do you fail to solve problems because you don't really *want* to exercise? If so, then do the following:

Focus on how you'll feel after you finish exercising, not on how you feel at the moment. Remind yourself that the hardest part is just getting started.

Put exercise in the NO CHOICE category. When you tell yourself, *I don't have time, I don't feel like it,* or *I don't want to,* respond the same way you've learned to respond to your cravings. Tell yourself that you don't have a choice. Tell yourself, *Oh, well,* and accept that you have to do it.

Meet a friend or trainer. At first, it might help to make an appointment with a friend or fitness professional or to sign up for a class. You'll be more likely to keep this commitment if you're accountable to someone. A trainer, fitness instructor, or knowledgeable friend can show you how to exercise properly, so you'll feel more confident that you're doing it correctly.

Give yourself lots of credit. Every small step in the right direction deserves credit. Reward yourself for exercising—just not with unplanned food!

Focus on your progress. Can you walk a minute longer than you used to? Can you exercise more vigorously than before? Remind yourself during every session that you're getting stronger and more physically fit.

End your session with something positive. If you like a particular piece of equipment or exercise, plan to do it last. If you dislike a part of your exercise routine, do it in the middle. This way, you'll leave feeling better about your exercise session and you'll be more likely to follow through and do it next time.

tip! If it's hard to make yourself exercise first thing in the morning, lay out your exercise clothes the night before. Tape Response Cards to your bathroom mirror. Remind yourself that your reluctance will disappear once you get started, and you'll be glad you got yourself to exercise.

Make sure you're doing a type of exercise you like. If you get bored with what you're doing, change it. One dieter told me that she finally hit on blasting music and strenuously dancing, all by herself, in her living room. Another dieter really disliked the exercise class she'd signed up for. She couldn't keep up. Finally, she switched to an easier class and began to enjoy it much more. A number of dieters have taken up organized sports instead of such solo exercise as running or swimming. Try out different possibilities.

what are you thinking?

The same types of thoughts that interfere with dieting can also interfere with exercising.

Sabotaging Thought: It's okay to skip exercising today because I don't want to, I'm tired, and I'm too stressed out.
Helpful Response: It's not okay. Exercise is an essential part of losing weight and maintaining my weight loss.

Sabotaging Thought: I'm not going to keep this up forever, so why start?
Helpful Response: I can do it today. If I have trouble doing it later on, I'll solve the problem then.

Sabotaging Thought: I'm not an exercise person.
Helpful Response: I don't have to be an exercise fanatic. I can continue doing what I've been doing and just gradually increase it, if I want to.

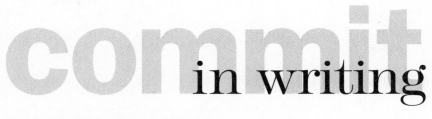

commit in writing

When I find myself resisting exercise, I'll: _____

_____

_____

_____

_____

_____

_____.

> Once I accept that exercise has
> to be a permanent part of my weight-loss
> program, dieting will be easier.

today's to-do list

Check off the tasks you've completed. For any item you haven't completed, record when you're going to complete it.

_____ I read my Advantages, NO CHOICE, It's Not Okay, Get Back on Track, and Believe It! Response Cards at least twice today.

_____ I read other Response Cards as needed.

_____ I ate slowly, sitting down and noticing every bite.

Circle one: Every time   Most of the time   Some of the time

_____ I gave myself credit for engaging in helpful eating behaviors.

Circle one: Every time   Most of the time   Some of the time

_____ I wrote a food plan for tomorrow and monitored everything I ate in writing right after I finished eating.

_____ I did spontaneous and planned exercise.

_____ I gave myself credit for exercising.

_____ I took steps to change my sabotaging thoughts about exercise.

day 40
Enrich Your Life

A lot of the dieters I counsel have the idea that they should put their lives on hold until they lose weight. Maggie is a good example. When I first started counseling her, we discussed how she thought her life would be different once she lost weight. She said that once she got to her goal, she wanted to go away for a vacation, buy a new wardrobe, start dating again (she was divorced), and look for a new job.

"Why don't you start doing some of those activities now?" I asked her.

Maggie looked puzzled. "You mean while I'm still heavy?"

"Yes, now. Why would you wait?" I inquired.

"Are you serious?" she asked. "I can't do those things now. It's because I want to be able to do these things that I'm dieting in the first place."

After our discussion, Maggie was able to see how enriching her life now could actually facilitate her weight loss. As she developed new interests, engaged in pleasurable activities, and felt more effective, her mood would lift, she'd focus on things other than food, and she'd have more mental energy to diet.

Like Maggie, have you put off enriching your life? Here's how to get started on making your life better today.

Do It *Now*

Put aside at least 10 minutes today during which you won't be interrupted or distracted. Then do the following:

- Take out your diet notebook. Make a list of goals that you'd like to accomplish before or after you lose weight. Do you want to change your job in some way? Become more computer savvy? Join a club? Meet new people? Improve relationships with family and friends? Pursue a hobby? Travel?
- Look at your list. See which of your "after weight loss" goals you could actually start working toward right away.
- Take one goal. Write down the steps you'll need to do to accomplish it.
- Get a calendar. Mark down when you'll do at least the first step.
- If you're uncertain of how to go about working toward a goal, ask friends or family for help. Mark on your calendar when you plan to consult with them. Doing so increases the likelihood that you'll go ahead and devise a plan.
- As you put activities on your calendar, watch for sabotaging thoughts. For example, if your goal is to look for a new job, you might think, *What if it doesn't work out?*

What if I don't like it? If your goal is to be more sociable, you might have such thoughts as, *What if no one wants to spend time with me?*

- Respond to your sabotaging thoughts in two ways: Look at the advantages and disadvantages of making this change in your life and use the Seven Question Technique on pages 199–203 to evaluate your concerns. Consult with your diet coach.
- Continue the process with a second goal.

Don't wait. Start engaging in some of these activities as soon as possible.

in session with Dr. Beck

Maggie is like many of the dieters I've worked with: She was embarrassed by her body. She hadn't put on a bathing suit in over three years. One day, she came in and told me that her best friend, Nina, had asked her if she wanted to go to the beach for a few days. Maggie was excited at the prospect of spending time with Nina, but she was very reluctant to reveal her body at the beach, even to her best friend. We had the following discussion.

Maggie: I know, I know, I really probably should go. On the other hand, I could wait till next summer when I'll be thinner.

Dr. Beck: Sure, you could do that. On the other hand, wouldn't it be better if you could get over your embarrassment?

Maggie: Probably.

Dr. Beck: Do you think you could picture yourself on the beach with Nina? What does Nina look like?

Maggie: Oh, she's probably a size 8 or 10. She looks fine.

Dr. Beck: And do you think you have an idea of what you'd look like—now? Not what you looked like before we started working together, but how you look now that you've lost 22 pounds?

Maggie: Well, I know I must look better than I did before. But people are going to see me and think, *Wow, she's a whale!*

Dr. Beck: Who's going to think that?

Maggie: Well, everyone on the beach.

Dr. Beck: Who do you think will be on the beach when you're there?

Maggie: Families, I guess. Teenagers. Maybe some people in their 20s. People of all ages, I guess.

Dr. Beck: Okay, the kids, how much attention will they be paying to you? Or will they be just running around, building sand castles, riding the waves ...

Maggie: I guess they might not notice me much.

Dr. Beck: And their parents? How much are they going to notice you versus how much are they going to be watching their kids?

Maggie: I guess they won't be noticing me much either.

Dr. Beck: Okay, now the teens and the people in their 20s and 30s. They might be looking around. Or they might be busy working on their suntans and talking to each other. If they do see you, they might think something unkind. How long do you think they'll be preoccupied with how you look?

Maggie: I'm not sure.

Dr. Beck: Okay, can we do an experiment together? We'll have to pretend that we're at the beach. You stay sitting in your chair, just pretend that it's a beach chair and that you're sitting under an umbrella with Nina, talking. Can you picture all of that in your mind?

Maggie: *[nods]*

Dr. Beck: *[gets up and sits on the floor about 10 feet behind her]* Here, I'm going to sit a little bit away from you. Okay, here's the scene. You and Nina are sitting in chairs, under the umbrella, you're talking, the sun is hot, maybe you're a little thirsty, you're enjoying facing the ocean and watching the people in the waves. Got it? Can you picture it?

Maggie: Yeah.

Dr. Beck: Okay, don't do it yet, but in a moment, you're going to turn your head and look at me. Pretend you're looking at someone who is about your size. When you do, keep looking at me for as long as you think an average person would. Then notice what you do next. Okay? Go!

Maggie: *[turns her head and looks at me and then looks away]* It wasn't that long, was it?

Dr. Beck: *[looks at watch]* No. It was four seconds. Why did you turn away and what did you do next?

Maggie: I was just thinking, *Wow, she's big!* But I guess I just wasn't too interested. Instead, I turned my head and looked at the ocean and started talking to my friend again.

Dr. Beck: Yes. *[pauses]* What does that tell you?

Maggie: I guess people probably won't spend much time thinking about me.

Dr. Beck: I think you're right. They're much more likely to be focusing on what interests them. My guess is that the only one your weight really interests is you.

Following our discussion, Maggie wrote the following Response Card:

It's really great that I'm here on the beach. It means I'm acting like a "normal" person. So what if I'm heavier than I want to be. I'm working on it. I've made a lot of progress so far. I'll get there. Meanwhile, it feels so good to feel the sun on me. It's so relaxing to watch the waves. And how wonderful it is to be here with Nina.

That night, Maggie made definite plans to go to the beach with Nina. She was also willing to start working toward some of her other goals. She finally recognized that there was no reason to wait to improve her life; she deserved to improve it right away.

what are you thinking?

You undoubtedly should enrich your life—now. Don't let the following sabotaging thoughts stop you.

Sabotaging Thought: I don't deserve to reward myself until I've lost all the weight I need to lose.
Helpful Response: Of course, I deserve to reward myself. Being overweight is not a moral failing. Everyone deserves to work toward having a better life.

Sabotaging Thought: I won't have as good a time if I [do this activity] before I've lost weight.
Helpful Response: That might be true, but before I go I can work on the unhelpful thoughts that could dampen my pleasure. I can [do this activity] once I lose weight, but I should also do it now. There's no reason to wait.

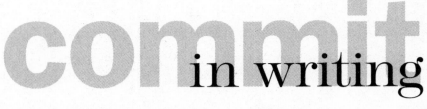

commit in writing

I'll schedule the first step of the following goals on my calendar: _____

_____

_____

_____

_____

_____

_____

_____.

Once I take steps to enrich
my life, dieting will be easier.

today's to-do list

Check off the tasks you've completed. For any item you haven't completed, record when you're going to complete it.

_____ I read my Advantages, NO CHOICE, It's Not Okay, Get Back on Track, and Believe It! Response Cards at least twice today.

_____ I read other Response Cards as needed.

_____ I ate slowly, sitting down and noticing every bite.

Circle one: Every time   Most of the time   Some of the time

_____ I gave myself credit for engaging in helpful eating behaviors.

Circle one: Every time   Most of the time   Some of the time

_____ I wrote a food plan for tomorrow and monitored everything I ate in writing right after I finished eating.

_____ I did spontaneous and planned exercise.

_____ I took steps to enrich my life.

day 41
Make a New To-Do List

You've now learned the skills you need to continue losing weight and to keep it off. You just have to keep practicing these skills—over and over and over—especially after you've reached your goal weight. In fact, you'll use some of the techniques for your entire life. Doing so is the key to continued success. The reason you regained weight in the past is that you didn't have these strategies. Now, you do.

Here are lists of techniques that you've learned, along with a guide for how often you should use them. I hope you've already found that you're doing some of these things automatically and that they've made dieting easier.

Do these activities daily:
- Eat a healthful diet with limited calories.
- Think about what you're eating before you actually put it in your mouth.
- Sit down whenever you eat and then eat slowly and mindfully.
- Eat only to mild fullness.
- Monitor your eating throughout the day.
- Give yourself credit.
- Do spontaneous exercise.
- Respond to sabotaging thoughts.

Do these activities between once a day and once a week:
- Weigh yourself at least once a week (daily, if you prefer).
- Discuss your weight change and dieting experiences with your diet coach at least once a week.
- Do planned exercise at least three times a week.
- Continue to make sure that you have enough time and energy to devote to dieting.
- Read your Advantages Response Card as needed.
- Use anti-craving techniques.
- Use the Seven Question Technique when you're upset.
- Prepare yourself psychologically for special-occasion eating.
- Do problem solving to reduce stress.
- Take steps to enrich your life.

Do these activities as often as needed (once a day, once a week, or less often, but certainly whenever you're in danger of straying from your diet):

Plan and monitor what you eat. Ideally, if you keep up one practice from this program for the rest of your life, this would be it. But if you find this task too burdensome, you can experiment with planning and monitoring in your head rather than writing down your food plan. Try it for a couple of days. If you do well, continue. But the moment you hit a rough patch—whenever you find yourself eating too much—start writing down what you plan to eat and monitor in writing what you actually do eat every day. DON'T GIVE YOURSELF A CHOICE ABOUT THIS.

You can also experiment with having a general plan about what you're going to eat and then decide before each meal what you're actually going to eat. For example, you might plan to have about a certain number of calories (or a certain portion size) of whatever protein, carbohydrates, and fat you want. But the moment you find yourself eating too much or not eating healthfully, go back to planning in advance. DON'T GIVE YOUR-SELF A CHOICE ABOUT THIS.

My experience has been that many people decide to stop writing down their food plans prematurely. They overestimate their ability to keep their eating in line without using this discipline. So don't be surprised if you find that you've stopped too soon. Don't get self-critical. Just go back to using this strategy when you need to.

Read your Response Cards. You've been reading some of your cards for almost six weeks. These responses are probably firmly in your mind. You can experiment with reading them on an as-needed basis. The moment you start to struggle, though, start reading them daily. DON'T GIVE YOUR-SELF A CHOICE ABOUT THIS.

what are you thinking?

Here are some sabotaging thoughts you might have. Use them to create your own Response Cards.

Sabotaging Thought: It's too much trouble to keep doing all these things.
Helpful Response: Losing weight is very important to me. It does take effort to do these things, but the payoff is tremendous.

Sabotaging Thought: I know what I'm supposed to do. I don't need to keep filling out the to-do list.
Helpful Response: What's the big deal? Better safe than sorry. I may as well assume I do need the list to motivate me and remind me what to do.

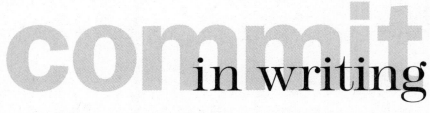

commit in writing

When I'm tempted to stop using the techniques on the to-do list, I'll: _____

_____

_____

_____

_____

_____

_____

_____

_____

_____

_____

_____.

> Once I create a consistent
> routine of using my weight-loss skills,
> dieting will be easier.

today's to-do list ...

... Is Also Your Future To-Do List

For the past six weeks, you've used a list at the end of each day to remind yourself what you need to do. Today's to-do list on the facing page is extensive. As described earlier in this chapter, you'll need to do some tasks on a daily or weekly basis and some just periodically.

To stay on track after today, you should fill out a to-do list every day for at least several weeks, then at least once a week for several weeks, and then monthly for a very long time. Start using it daily again if you find that you're becoming lax in your eating or exercising or if you begin to struggle to get yourself to do what you know you need to do.

As always, whenever you fill out a to-do list, check off the items you've completed. For any item you haven't completed, record when you're going to complete it.

_____ I read my Advantages, NO CHOICE, It's Not Okay, Get Back on Track, and Believe It! Response Cards as needed.

_____ I read my other Response Cards as needed.

_____ I wrote out a food plan for tomorrow.

_____ I monitored everything I ate in writing right after I finished eating.

_____ I talked to my diet coach.

_____ Every time I ate, I sat down and ate slowly and mindfully.

_____ I ate only to mild fullness.

_____ I gave myself credit whenever I engaged in helpful eating behaviors.

_____ I removed or rearranged tempting food in my home and work environments.

_____ I changed my schedule to increase my time and energy for dieting.

_____ I took steps to reduce stress.

_____ I did spontaneous exercise at every opportunity.

_____ I did planned exercise.

_____ I reminded myself that hunger is never an emergency.

_____ I tolerated a craving or used anti-craving techniques rather than giving in.

_____ If I overate or strayed from my diet, I got back on track immediately.

_____ I said, *Oh, well,* or *NO CHOICE,* whenever I wanted to eat something I wasn't supposed to.

_____ I responded effectively to ideas of unfairness and discouragement.

_____ I used the Seven Question Technique to respond to my sabotaging thoughts and made corresponding Response Cards.

_____ When others offered me food that I hadn't planned to eat, I turned them down.

_____ I followed my diet successfully when I ate out.

_____ I experienced negative emotion and didn't turn to food for comfort.

_____ I took steps to enrich my life.

_____ I prepared myself for weighing in.

day 42
Practice, Practice, Practice

Congratulations! You've learned the Cognitive Therapy skills you need to think like a thin person. The longer you use these new thinking skills, the more automatic they'll become. Dieting will continue to get easier and easier. Do you remember the differences in thinking between naturally thin people and people who struggle with dieting, which were described on pages 34–41? Your thinking has fundamentally changed in the past six weeks. If you ever find yourself slipping back to your old way of thinking, review "Reminders to Think Thin" on the facing page.

Remember that you'll hit rough patches from time to time. All dieters occasionally give in to cravings, forget to give themselves credit, or neglect to follow their food plan. All dieters occasionally question whether losing weight is worth the time and effort. Whenever you hit a rough patch, go back to this book. Flip through each day of the program, reread the passages you need, and start doing the relevant tasks again.

Also, recognize that rough patches are TEMPORARY. You'll soon be glad that you persevered, especially as you're getting compliments, fitting into clothes you couldn't fit in before, and seeing the number on the scale go down. I promise you that even if it doesn't feel worth it at any given moment, it *will* soon!

The next two chapters are just as important as the ones you've just finished. You'll learn how to determine a comfortable weight that you can successfully maintain for a very long time and what you need to do to make sure you can sustain that weight. Once you finish these chapters, you can feel confident that you now think and behave like a thin person—and will continue to do so for the rest of your life!

reminders to think thin

If you think ... *I hadn't planned to eat this food, but I'm hungry. I have to eat right now!*

Remind yourself ... Barring a medical problem, I don't *need* to eat. I just *want* to eat. But I want all the benefits of weight loss much more than I want the momentary pleasure of eating.

If you think ... *Even though I've finished everything on my plate, I want to keep eating. I like feeling really full.*

Remind yourself ... Trying to become overly full is a habit that is likely to lead to weight gain. I need to stop when the food I've planned to eat is gone. My hunger will subside within 20 minutes.

If you think ... *It's okay to eat this [unplanned food] because: everyone else is eating it; it'll go to waste; it was free; I'm celebrating; I'm upset; I really want it; I don't care; it won't matter.*

Remind yourself ... It's not okay to eat this; I'm just trying to fool myself. Every single time I eat something I'm not supposed to, I strengthen my giving-in muscle and weaken my resistance muscle.

If you think ... *I can't believe the scale has gone up! This is terrible! I'll never be able to lose weight.*

Remind yourself ... My weight is supposed to go up sometimes. I should continue with the Beck Diet Solution program and wait two weeks before assuming there is a problem.

If you think ... *It's not fair that I can't eat normally and have what everyone else is eating.*

Remind yourself ... I'm now eating normally for a person who has a goal to lose weight. It would be even more unfair if I let feelings of unfairness keep me from becoming thinner.

If you think ... *Now that I've lost weight, I can stop being so careful.*

Remind yourself ... If I want to keep the weight off, I need to use the techniques I've learned for the rest of my life. If I don't continue to maintain my new mindset and eating behaviors, I'll invariably gain back weight.

Going Forward

chapter 11

When to Stop Losing and Start Maintaining

W hen should you stop dieting and start rest-of-your-life eating? That's not an easy question to answer. It's not just a matter of getting down to a predetermined goal you've set for yourself because that weight might or might not be realistic for you to achieve or to maintain. In fact, when I meet with dieters for the first time, I ask them two questions:

1. What would you like to weigh? (In other words, what is your ideal goal?)
2. What weight could make you at least minimally satisfied? (In other words, what is your satisfaction goal?)

It's always a good sign when the numbers aren't identical. It means that those dieters are probably more realistic about what they can accomplish than dieters who give me numbers that are the same.

For example, Julia, who started at 175 pounds, told me that her ideal goal was 120 pounds and that her satisfaction goal was 130 pounds. She actually has maintained her weight for more than 10 years at 128 pounds (plus or minus 2 pounds)—quite happily. On the other hand, Christine, who started at 136 pounds, said she ideally wanted to get down to 115 pounds but would be satisfied with 118 pounds. She was initially disappointed when I told her we wouldn't know for a while whether her range was realistic or not. In fact, she was able to get down to 120 pounds and has maintained at about 124 pounds for five years. It took her a while to accept this as her reasonable maintenance weight.

So how do you know when you've reached maintenance? How can you determine a realistic maintenance weight? You'll find a formula in the following pages. But, first, you need to understand the difference between your Lowest Achievable Weight and your Lowest Maintainable Weight.

Your Lowest Achievable Weight Versus Your Lowest Maintainable Weight

Let's say you've been slowly losing weight while eating a fairly consistent number of calories each day and getting about the same amount of exercise each week. At some point, your weight will naturally plateau, even though you aren't doing anything differently. If your weight remains constant for several weeks, you'll have to make a decision, as described on page 248: You can continue as is and see what happens; or, if it's reasonable to do so, you can cut your food intake by about 200 calories a day (if your health-care professional agrees) or increase your exercise and see what happens.

At some point, though, you'll stop losing weight and it will no longer be sensible for you to decrease your caloric intake or to increase your exercise. You've reached your Lowest Achievable Weight.

Your **LOWEST ACHIEVABLE WEIGHT** *is the weight at which you naturally plateau.*

You might not be able to stay at your Lowest Achievable Weight, however, because to do so you would have to keep on eating the same number of calories and exercising to the same degree for the rest of your life. In fact,

> *At some point, you'll stop losing weight* **and it will no longer be sensible for you to decrease your caloric intake or to increase your exercise.**

as you age, your metabolism will slow, and you'll have to decrease your caloric intake or increase your energy output even more to maintain that weight. It just might not be reasonable to expect yourself to stay at your Lowest Achievable Weight forever.

Instead, you should consider raising your number of calories modestly or decreasing your exercise (if you feel you're overdoing it in order to maintain your Lowest Achievable Weight) to a level you can more easily adhere to. Your weight will probably go up a little, but it will plateau again at your Lowest Maintainable Weight.

Your **LOWEST MAINTAINABLE WEIGHT** *is the weight you can sustain permanently, while still following a sensible eating and exercise program for the rest of your life.*

Your Lowest Maintainable Weight might not be the lowest weight you've ever been in your adult life. Maybe you weighed significantly less at some point because your lifestyle was different, you were much more physically active, you'd been sick, or you were younger and had a higher metabolism. Even if you could achieve this weight again, you most likely would not be able to maintain this weight.

Your Lowest Maintainable Weight also is probably not the weight of your thinnest friend, family member, neighbor, coworker, or person you see at the gym. And it almost certainly is not the weight of celebrities or fashion models, who eat an incredibly (usually quite unhealthy) low number of calories a day and spend hours and hours exercising.

Determine Your Lowest Achievable Weight

When your weight plateaus for a month or two, think about your caloric intake. Ask yourself:

- *Do I want to reduce my calories even more?*
- *Will I get enough satisfaction from eating if I eat less?*
- *Will eating even less still be healthy?*
- *Will eating less fit into my lifestyle?*
- *Could I comfortably live with a reduced number of calories for the long term?*

If you answered yes to all these questions, then cut your calories modestly (by about 200 calories a day) and see if you lose weight.

You can also think about exercising more. Ask yourself:

- *Do I really want to increase the frequency, intensity, or duration of my exercise?*
- *Will I have enough extra time and energy to devote to more exercise?*
- *Will exercising more be healthy for me—or will I be overdoing it?*
- *Will I easily be able to keep up an increased level of exercise for the long term?*

If you answered yes to all those questions, then increase your exercise modestly and see what happens.

If you lose more weight by eating less or exercising more, fine. Keep up with your new routine until you reach a new plateau and reassess the situation.

When Gina, a teacher, plateaued for several weeks at 132 pounds, she wanted to keep losing. She thought she'd be able to cut her calories and exercise more. But when we analyzed her situation, it became apparent that she could do so only for a couple of months, during her summer off from teaching. When she returned to school in September, she knew she'd have less control over her schedule and food. She reluctantly agreed that it didn't make sense to try to lose a few more pounds, since she'd likely regain them within a short period of time.

Determine Your Lowest Maintainable Weight

Let's say that you've plateaued at your Lowest Achievable Weight for several weeks or months. Then you realize that the strict eating and exercise routine you've been following to stay there is too much of a struggle. Maybe you feel hungry or deprived too frequently. Maybe you'd like to be able to eat out more or drink wine with dinner. Maybe you have less control over your eating schedule or choice of foods. Maybe your lifestyle has changed, and you simply can't devote as much time and energy to food preparation or exercise. It's not that you're less motivated; there really are obstacles in your way.

At this point, make a decision to eat a little bit more or decide to exercise a little less. You need an eating and exercise plan you can comfortably live with for the rest of your life. Rather than just drifting into changes in your routines, sit down (preferably with your diet coach) and write a new plan in your diet notebook. How many extra calories do you want to consume per day or per week? How much do you need to cut back on exercise?

You need an eating and exercise plan you can comfortably live with for the rest of your life.

Follow this plan for several months, revising it as needed. You'll gain a few pounds and plateau again. This is your Lowest Maintainable Weight. You may find that this initial Lowest Maintainable Weight works well for several years. As your metabolism slows with age, you might need to reset your Lowest Maintainable Weight. The weight that you maintain at one age may or may not be a reasonable weight to maintain 10 years later. Don't allow yourself to just drift to a higher weight, though. When you gain, make sure it isn't because you've become lax in your eating habits or exercise routine. If you want to be able to eat the same amount or if you want to be able to eat a little more, set a new Lowest Maintainable Weight, a weight you'll not let yourself go beyond.

But I Want to Be Thinner!

This is a statement I hear a lot. You recognize that you've reached your Lowest Maintainable Weight, but you don't want to accept it. You really want to be thinner. You're thinking, *I don't like how I look at this weight.* You can do a number of things if you're unhappy with your Lowest Maintainable Weight.

Continue to enrich your life. If you haven't already, it's now time to do all the things you put off until you lost weight, as discussed on Day 40 (pages 256–260). The richer your social, family, work, spiritual, intellectual, creative, and recreational life, the less you'll focus on your weight. Compared to these important aspects of your experience, the desire to be even thinner is really superficial, isn't it?

Focus on the parts of your body that please you the most. I'll bet your automatic tendency is to focus on the parts of your body that you don't like. Of course, you're going to feel dissatisfied. Instead, focus on the parts that you *do* like.

Say to yourself, *Oh, well.* Think about how you've been able to accept a lesser goal in other parts of your life. How did you come to peace with it? Do you still struggle every day because your job isn't as satisfying as you want, your home doesn't look the way you'd like it to, you don't have as much time as you'd like for recreational activities? Or have you come to accept these imperfections in your life? Have you said, *Oh, well, I'm not crazy about this aspect of my life, but I guess I can't have everything ... and I'm glad that I at least have [e.g., good friends, a good job, a hobby I love]*? You might need to do the same with your weight.

Focus on how you've improved. You might not be as thin as you'd like, but how many of the benefits of weight loss have you achieved? Do you look better than you used to? Do you get more compliments? Are you wearing different clothes? Do you have more self-confidence? Do you feel more in control? Do you feel better about yourself? Do you have more energy? Are you healthier? Do you feel less self-conscious? Focusing on all the benefits you've derived instead of on an unrealistic number on the scale will make you feel better.

Change your comparison. If you compare yourself with people who weigh less than you or if you compare yourself to what you wish you weighed, you'll always be unhappy. Change the comparison. Contrast how you look today with how you looked when you first started this program.

Prepare yourself mentally before you weigh yourself. You'll feel disappointed if you continually expect to see your Lowest Achievable Weight whenever you step on the scale. Before you weigh yourself, remind yourself of your Lowest Maintainable Weight. Also remind yourself that you'll probably weigh between 2 pounds more to 2 pounds less than that number. This way, you'll be happy, rather than disappointed, when the scale shows that you've maintained. If you gain more than 2 pounds, tell yourself that you now have the skills to solve the problem.

> ## The richer your life, *the less you'll focus on your weight.*

Accept compliments from others. When others tell you how wonderful you look, you might silently say to yourself, *But I should look better.* If so, make sure to respond to that sabotaging thought. Try to see things from the speakers' points of view. They're not thinking you should look even better. They're just thinking you look good. And if you don't already respond to such compliments graciously, make sure to always thank people without any qualification. Don't say, "Thank you, but...." Just say, "Thank you."

Act "as if." Imagine how you'd think, feel, and act if you were currently at your ideal weight. As you go through the day, pretend you are at that weight. If you do, chances are that you'll stand a little taller, be less self-conscious, and project greater self-confidence. If you continually act "as if," you'll eventually stop pretending and gradually become more satisfied.

You might instantly be able to accept your Lowest Maintainable Weight without struggle. Or you might have to do the tasks above to increase your acceptance over time. Work at it. Discuss it with your friends and diet coach. What a shame if you can't fully enjoy your new body and you continue to go through life feeling dissatisfied. How wonderful it will be when you stop struggling and feel really good about where you are.

in session with Dr. Beck

When Ellen started working with me, she was 5'3" and weighed 145 pounds. Despite our discussions, she harbored a hope all along that she'd be able to get down to 114 pounds, a pound lighter than her older sister. With considerable effort, she reached 114 pounds and stayed there—for about three days. Then she moved up to 116, where she stayed, more or less, for about three months. At that point, she got a new job, which required that she sit at a desk. She made some new friends and began to have a better social life, going out several nights a week. Her weight rose during the next eight weeks to 120 pounds. But it stayed there—it became her Lowest Maintainable Weight. She had to work toward accepting that weight, so we had the following discussion.

Ellen: But I don't like weighing 120. I don't think I look thin enough.

Dr. Beck: I know you don't. And you're feeling disappointed.

Ellen: Yeah. I don't know if I can accept it.

Dr. Beck: Ellen, what are the advantages of holding onto this hope that you can be thinner?

Ellen: *[thinks]* None, I guess.

Dr. Beck: And what are the disadvantages?

Ellen: *[glumly]* I guess it makes me unhappy.

Dr. Beck: I think you're right. As another example, what if you had a goal to win an Olympic medal? And you realized every day that that was just not going to happen.

Ellen: I'd feel bad, of course.

Dr. Beck: Do you have that as a goal?

Ellen: *[laughs]* No.

Dr. Beck: So do you feel bad about it every day?

Ellen: No.

Dr. Beck: So, as long as you can't achieve it, it's good that you're not aiming toward it. Is that right?

Ellen: Yeah, I guess so.

Dr. Beck: So how does that relate to this idea of trying to get down to and stay at 114 pounds?

Ellen: *[sighs]* I guess if that's my goal, I'm going to stay unhappy.

Dr. Beck: Okay, now let's say, hypothetically, that you were able to change your goal to be 120 pounds. How would you feel every day when you got on the scale?

Ellen: Well, better, I guess.

Dr. Beck: So how would you like to feel for the rest of your life: bad or better?

Ellen: Well, better, of course.

Dr. Beck: So that means ...

Ellen: *[sighs]* That I have to change my goal.

Dr. Beck: And as long as you don't accept this? As long as you keep trying for something that's not realistic?

Ellen: I'll feel bad. *[pauses]* But I still feel a little bad that I can't have 114 as my goal.

Next, I helped Ellen see that her life wouldn't be any different if she weighed less. And she was able to recognize that everyone else thinks she looks good at her current weight.

Dr. Beck: So maybe the problem isn't that you can't maintain at 114 pounds. Maybe the problem is what you tell yourself when you look in the mirror. Did you look in the mirror this morning?

Ellen: Sure.

Dr. Beck: And what went through your mind?

Ellen: I was thinking my stomach looks too big.

Dr. Beck: Which made you feel ...

Ellen: Bad.

Dr. Beck: What if you'd thought, *Wow, look at me ... I look so different from how I did five months ago ... This is great!*

Ellen: I'd feel better.

Dr. Beck: So you have a choice: You can struggle with yourself about weighing 120 and keep telling yourself that you don't look good enough, or you can say, *Oh, well, this is my Lowest Maintainable Weight ... Check out how good I look compared to before.*

Ellen made a Response Card, highlighting these new ideas, which she read every morning before she got dressed and looked in her full-length mirror.

It's wonderful that I've lost weight. I should celebrate the "new me," not cricitize myself. I don't look perfect, but I look much better and feel much better. It's great to be at this new weight.

chapter 12

How to Stay at Your New Weight

The first thing I want you to do when you reach your Lowest Maintainable Weight is give yourself lots of credit. It's wonderful you got to this point! Did you think when you first picked up this book that you'd really get here? Well, you have! It's a major accomplishment—you should be very proud of yourself. Okay, now you need to learn how to stay there:

Continue to weigh yourself between once a day and once a week. All the maintainers I've worked with found that they needed to be vigilant about their weight. The only surefire method is to habitually use the scale. Those who stopped weighing themselves usually did fine for a period of time (months to years), but eventually they started gaining again.

Recommit yourself if you gain 3 pounds. Three pounds seems to be the magic number according to the maintainers I've counseled because if they went 3 pounds above their Lowest Maintainable Weight, they were likely to continue gaining. If you gain 3 pounds, you don't have to do every task in the program, but I do advise you to reread the program days in this book to see which skills you should reinstate. Sometimes, it's just a matter of putting a plan in writing, measuring your food, and monitoring what you're eating for a couple of weeks.

Create a Maintenance Advantages Response Card. Create a new card that reflects all the reasons that you don't want to regain weight. Use the Advantages Response Card you created before you started to lose weight for help in creating your card for maintenance. What benefits of weight loss have come true for you? Have you experienced additional unexpected advantages that you hadn't written on your card? List all of these on your new card, after the following sentence: "I want to maintain my weight loss because I want to continue to...." Pull it out when you need it, whenever you're tempted to eat more or exercise less.

Anticipate the amount of effort required for maintenance. Have you heard that it's harder to maintain your weight loss than it is to lose it initially? I've not found this to be true among the dieters I've worked with. The course of maintenance frequently follows the same course as dieting. It's easier in the beginning, at some point it gets more difficult, and then it gets easier again. It stays easier most of the time, with intermittent periods when it's more difficult. It's important for you to have this expectation, or you'll be disappointed when maintenance occasionally requires more effort. If you don't realize that this is normal, you might get discouraged, put in less effort, and then regain weight. Make yourself a Response Card to remind yourself that maintenance is supposed to be hard at times, but that it *will* get easier again.

Give yourself credit multiple times a day for using all of your behavioral and mindset skills.

Respond to any sabotaging thoughts. Expect to have sabotaging thoughts periodically for a very long time. You'll get better and better at responding to them, but you'll need to pull out your Response Cards whenever you're having difficulty. I'd also like you to read them periodically, even if you don't think it's necessary. Most of the maintainers I work with read their cards

can I just listen to my body?

When many dieters reach maintenance, they ask me whether they can stop following a plan and instead follow their natural hunger cues, eating when they feel hungry and stopping once they feel full. I personally have never worked with a maintainer who could use hunger as a guide instead of planning what he or she is going to eat or sticking to a general routine of meals and snacks. If you want to try, it's probably better to wait quite a while because you might still have a tendency to mislabel a desire or craving as hunger. When you do try, watch the scale. If you regain weight, go back to planning.

weekly when they first reach maintenance, then once every two weeks, then once a month, and then once every season. Remember to use the Seven Question Technique (pages 199–203) and create a new Response Card whenever you identify new sabotaging thoughts.

Eat the same amount of food and same number of calories that you've been eating as you stabilized your weight. If you find that you want to eat more, make a conscious decision to set a new Lowest Maintainable Weight.

Continue to plan and monitor what you eat. As you learned on Day 41 (pages 261–265), at some point you can experiment with planning and monitoring mentally. Even if you're not writing down a specific food plan, though, you'll need to have a general plan of what you're going to eat each day. After a while, you might be able to get to the point where you don't necessarily need to decide the night before what you're going to have for each snack or meal. You know you'll most likely choose from among your regular menus.

Create menus. Research shows that successful maintainers tend to eat many of the same foods from day to day. Most of the maintainers I've worked with have about three different breakfast and lunch menus and about eight different dinner and snack menus. They don't limit themselves to these menus, but they eat these meals most of the time. Having limited options makes life easier. You know which kinds of food can keep you at your Lowest Maintainable Weight. And you know which foods you'll need to shop for every week and how long it will take to prepare each meal.

Eat consistently day to day. Research also shows that you're more likely to maintain your weight if you don't vary your caloric intake significantly from one day to the next. That means that you might eat more on special occasions but not a *lot* more. And you won't vary much whether it's a weekend or a weekday.

Use good eating habits. Make sure you continually eat slowly, while sitting down, noticing every bite, and stopping when you're just mildly full.

Keep up with exercise. This means both spontaneous and planned, at least to the same degree as when you reached your Lowest Maintainable Weight. If your circumstances change and you need to exercise less, you might have to adjust your Lowest Maintainable Weight. Exercise is often one of the first things to drop off people's to-do list when they get busy. But research shows that it's an essential part of maintenance. Don't let yourself go more than a week (two at the most) without doing planned exercise. Do spontaneous exercise every day, no matter what.

Continue to get support. Even at the maintenance phase, it's important to check in periodically with your diet coach and report the status of your weight, if for no other reason than to keep yourself honest. In addition, your coach can help you solve problems and offer emotional support during stressful times. Both will prevent you from reverting to eating as a coping strategy. Even when you're not feeling particularly stressed, you might need occasional help in continuing to create enough time and energy to maintain your weight.

Consider becoming a diet coach. One of the best ways to keep your skills sharp is to teach them to someone else.

Take pleasure in your weight loss and in your level of fitness. Remind yourself every day how much you enjoy being thinner, healthier, and more physically fit—and how much you want to stay this way.

Keep in Touch!

I'd really like to hear about your successes or difficulties following the Beck Diet Solution. I'd also like to know what strategies and tips you have that I didn't include in this book.

Please write to me online by visiting **www.beckdietsolution.com** or send a letter to me at Beck Institute for Cognitive Therapy, P.O. Box 2673, Bala Cynwyd, PA 19004.

As I learn more from you, from other dieters, and from researchers, I'll update the Web site and fill you in.

BEST OF LUCK!
Judith Beck

Selected Bibliography

The Power of Cognitive Therapy for Weight Loss

Dansinger, M.; Augustin, J.; Griffith, J.; Selker, H.; Schaefer, E. "Comparison of the Atkins, Ornish, Weight Watchers, and Zone Diets for Weight Loss and Heart Disease Risk Reduction." *Journal of the American Medical Association*. Vol. 293, No. 1 (January 2005): 43–53.

Foster, G.D.; Makris, A.P.; Bailer, B.A. "Behavioral Treatment of Obesity." *American Journal of Clinical Nutrition*. Vol. 82, Supplement 1 (July 2005): 230S–235S.

Paykel, E.S.; Scott, J.; Teasdale, J.D.; Johnson, A.L.; Garland, A.; Moore, R.; Jenaway, A.; Cornwall, P.L.; Hayhurst, H.; Abbott, R.; Pope, M. "Prevention of Relapse in Residual Depression by Cognitive Therapy: A Controlled Trial." *Archives of General Psychiatry*. Vol. 56, No. 9 (September 1999): 829–835.

Stahre, L.; Hallstrom, T. "A Short-Term Cognitive Group Treatment Program Gives Substantial Weight Reduction Up to 18 Months from the End of Treatment. A Randomized Controlled Trial." *Eating and Weight Disorders*. Vol. 10, No. 1: 51–58.

The Program

Baker, R.C.; Kirschenbaum, D.S. "Weight Control During the Holidays: Highly Consistent Self-Monitoring as a Potentially Useful Coping Mechanism." *Health Psychology*. Vol. 17, No. 4 (July 1998): 367–370.

Burke, L.E.; Sereika, S.; Choo, J.; Warziski, M.; Music, E.; Styn, M.; Novak, J.; Stone, A. "Ancillary Study to the PREFER Trial: A Descriptive Study of Participants' Patterns of Self-Monitoring—Rationale, Design and Preliminary Experiences." *Contemporary Clinical Trials*. Vol. 27, No. 1 (February 2006): 23–33.

Carels, R.A.; Darby, L.A.; Rydin, S.; Douglass, O.M.; Cacciapaglia, H.M.; O'Brien, W.H. "The Relationship Between Self-Monitoring, Outcome Expectancies, Difficulties with Eating and Exercise, and Physical Activity and Weight Loss Treatment Outcomes." *Annals of Behavioral Medicine*. Vol. 30, No. 3 (December 2005): 182–190.

Green, M.W.; Elliman, N.A.; Kretsch, M.J. "Weight Loss Strategies, Stress, and Cognitive Function: Supervised Versus Unsupervised Dieting." *Psychoneuroendocrinology*. Vol. 30, No. 9 (October 2005): 908–918.

Harvey-Berino, J.; Pintauro, S.; Buzzell, P.; Gold, E.C. "Effect of Internet Support on the Long-Term Maintenance of Weight Loss." *Obesity Research*. Vol. 12, No. 2 (February 2004): 320–329.

Jones, K.L.; O'Donovan, D.; Horowitz, M.; Russo, A.; Lei, Y.; Hausken, T. "Effects of Posture on Gastric Emptying, Transpyloric Flow, and Hunger After a Glucose Drink in Healthy Humans." *Digestive Diseases and Sciences*. Vol. 51, No. 8 (August 2006): 1331–1338.

Marjorie, R.; Freedman, M.; King, J.; Kennedy, E. "Popular Diets: A Scientific Review." *Obesity Research*. Vol. 9, Supplement: 1S–5S.

Martin, C. "Does Slower Eating Rate Reduce Food Intake? Results of an Empirical Test," presented at the North American Association for the Study of Obesity 2004 Annual Scientific Meeting, Nov. 14–18, 2004, Las Vegas, Nevada.

Pendleton, V.R.; Goodrick, G.K.; Poston, W.S.; Reeves, R.S.; Foreyt, J.P. "Exercise Augments the Effects of Cognitive-Behavioral Therapy in the Treatment of Binge Eating." *The International Journal of Eating Disorders*. Vol. 31, No. 2 (March 2002): 172–184.

Procidano, M.; Heller, K. "Measures of Perceived Social Support from Friends and from Family: Three Validation Studies." *American Journal of Community Psychology*. Vol. 11, No. 1 (February 1983): 1–24.

Rolls, B.J.; Roe, L.S.; Meengs, J.S. "Larger Portion Sizes Lead to a Sustained Increase in Energy Intake Over 2 days." *Journal of the American Dietetic Association*. Vol. 106, No. 4 (April 2006): 543–549.

Wansink, B. "Ice Cream Illusions Bowls, Spoons, and Self-Served Portion Sizes." *American Journal of Preventive Medicine*. Vol. 31, No. 3 (September 2006): 240–243.

Wing, R.R.; Jeffery, R.W. "Benefits of Recruiting Participants with Friends and Increasing Social Support for Weight Loss and Maintenance." *Journal of Consulting and Clinical Psychology*. Vol. 67, No. 1 (February 1999): 132–138.

Going Forward

Wing, R.; Phelan, S. "Long-Term Weight Maintenance." *American Journal of Clinical Nutrition*. Vol. 82, No. 1, Supplement (July 2005): 222S–225S.

Index